Nutrition at a Glance

Nutrition at a Glance

Mary E. Barasi BA, BSc, MSc, RNutr

Principal Lecturer in Nutrition,
University of Wales Institute,
Cardiff

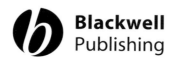
Blackwell Publishing

Blackwell Publishing editorial offices:
Blackwell Publishing Ltd, 9600 Garsington Road, Oxford OX4 2DQ, UK
Tel: +44 (0)1865 776868
Blackwell Publishing Inc., 350 Main Street, Malden, MA 02148-5020, USA
Tel: +1 781 388 8250
Blackwell Publishing Asia Pty Ltd, 550 Swanston Street, Carlton, Victoria 3053, Australia
Tel: +61 (0)3 8359 1011

First published 2007 by Blackwell Publishing Ltd

ISBN: 9781405134873

Library of Congress Cataloging-in-Publication Data
Barasi, Mary E.
  Nutrition at a glance / Mary E. Barasi.
    p. ; cm. -- (At a glance series)
  Includes index.
  ISBN-13: 978-1-4051-3487-3 (pbk. : alk. paper)
  ISBN-10: 1-4051-3487-9 (pbk. : alk. paper) 1. Nutrition--Handbooks, manuals, etc. I. Title. II. Series: At
a glance series (Oxford, England)
  [DNLM: 1. Nutrition Physiology--Handbooks. 2. Nutrition Disorders--Handbooks. QU 39 B225n 2007]

  QP141.A1B3776 2007
  612.3--dc22

                                                                    2007003617

A catalogue record for this title is available from the British Library

Set in 9.5 on 12pt Times by Sparks – www.sparks.co.uk
Printed and bound in Singapore by Markono Print Media Pte Ltd

For further information on Blackwell Publishing, visit our website:
www.blackwellpublishing.com

Contents

1 Diet, health and disease

Aims

(1) To gain a perspective on some of the links between diet, health and disease.

(2) To recognise the complexity of some relationships between diet, health and disease.

(3) To start to recognise the role of nutritional epidemiology in the study of such relationships.

A healthy diet and lifestyle are generally recognised as prerequisites for health, defined as the promotion of quality of life, or wellness, and the prevention of nutrition-related disease.

Identifying specific components of diet and lifestyle that can ensure health remains a challenge, as the relationships are complex. Scientific approaches, such as nutritional epidemiology, can provide evidence on which advice and policy can be based. Developments parallel advances in scientific methodology, which allow new approaches to be used in nutritional studies.

Historical perspective

Early studies in nutrition originated from observations of deficiency diseases, for which the cure with a single nutrient was eventually discovered. This led the way to the identification of many of the micronutrients. (see Table 1.1). Examples include:

• Scurvy was observed in sailors on long sea voyages and was treated in the eighteenth century with citrus fruits. It was not identified as a vitamin C deficiency until the early twentieth century, when the guinea pig was found to be susceptible to the deficiency.

• Beri-beri, the deficiency of thiamin, was discovered in Java, in humans and birds fed polished rice; it could be cured by feeding the rice bran, which was eventually shown to be rich in the vitamin.

• The association between low levels of iodine in food and drinking water and the swelling of the thyroid gland, known as goitre, was described in the early nineteenth century. However, the key role of iodine in the formation of thyroid hormones was not elucidated until the early part of the twentieth century.

• Iron, folate and vitamin B_{12} deficiencies are associated with anaemias that have distinct cytological pictures. Although the common feature was anaemia, its origin involved different dietary patterns, and required differential diagnosis and treatments.

• Some relationships proved to involve several factors, e.g. the development of rickets as a result of vitamin D deficiency. Although it can be obtained in the diet, for most people synthesis in the skin on exposure to sunlight is the most important source of the vitamin. Exposure to 'country air', out of smoky cities, was believed initially to be the cure. More recently it has also been shown that hydroxylation of the vitamin takes place in the liver and kidney, to produce the active form, so an association with disease in these organs also causes the deficiency. Additional roles for vitamin D in cellular metabolism have now been described.

More lessons about the link between diet and disease have been learned from instances of toxicity resulting from overconsumption of dietary factors. Classic examples include:

• Toxic effects from excess intake of vitamin A were recorded in polar explorers consuming the liver of polar bears. More recently, excessive intake of vitamin A, often as a supplement, has been shown to cause fetal malformations in early pregnancy, and may cause bone fractures.

• Hypercalcaemia in infants in the early 1950s resulted from excessive intakes of formula milk and cod-liver oil supplements containing large amounts of vitamin D.

• Excessive intakes of alcohol over time are known to cause liver damage, but the exact aetiology of this toxic effect is likely to be multifactorial, involving other dietary changes consequent on alcohol consumption.

Once the link between a nutrient and disease was established, public health measures were introduced to treat the condition.

Table 1.1 Examples of nutrition-related disease predominantly associated with single dietary factors.

Disease/abnormality	Dietary factor
Deficiency	
Scurvy	Vitamin C
Beri-beri	Thiamin
Goitre	Iodine
Rickets	Vitamin D
Anaemias	Iron/folate/vitamin B_{12}
Overconsumption	
Fetal abnormalities	Vitamin A
Infant hypercalcaemia	Vitamin D
Liver cirrhosis	Alcohol

Simple measures to rectify deficiencies of individual nutrients

• Parboiling of rice before it is milled ensures that some of the thiamin in the husk is transferred into the grain and improves its thiamin content.

• In iodine-deficient areas the addition of iodine to common salt ensures that a frequently used commodity provides the missing nutrient, and reduces the burden of deficiency.

• When formula milk was introduced in the UK for infant feeding, it was fortified with vitamins A and D. The level of vitamin D was initially excessive (see above). Present-day infant milks are carefully formulated to provide nutrients in amounts that match those in human milk.

• Women of child-bearing age who might become pregnant are advised to take a folic acid supplement as a measure to reduce the risk of neural-tube defects (NTD) in the infant. This is not based on traditional deficiency studies but on evidence from trials showing that such supplementation does reduce the risk of NTD. In the USA, grain products are supplemented with folate, and there has been a significant reduction in NTD cases. This measure is now being considered in the UK.

Several dietary factors implicated in disease

In some diseases, the role of individual dietary components is difficult to identify. Ongoing research adds further understanding, but also raises more questions. This can be illustrated for cardiovascular disease and cancer (see Box).

Other factors affecting susceptibility to disease

Dietary factors do not operate in isolation, their effects are modified or amplified by fixed or changeable factors, including:

- genetic susceptibility;
- aspects of early life in the uterine environment;
- environmental factors in the individual's life;
- lifestyle.

Even for a condition, such as overweight, that has an apparently simple cause (excessive energy intake in relation to output), the exact mechanisms involved and the ways to intervene for any one individual are not easy to find.

All of these interlinking factors make it very difficult to:

- identify precisely the role of any single dietary component;
- formulate policy to advise on and influence change.

Further, it should be recognised that in the diet–health–disease relationship, different factors may be involved in the *initiation* of the disease and others in the *progression* of the disease. Disease *prevention* may involve yet other factors and these limitations must be taken into account in the formulation of public health advice.

Introduction to nutritional epidemiology

(1) This is the major scientific method for the study of the relationship between exposure to particular dietary factors and the outcome in terms of causation or prevention of disease; it investigates the strength of such relationships.

(2) It cannot, however, establish a definitive cause for an outcome.

(3) A number of established standards (see Box) must be fulfilled before any conclusions about causality can be drawn. The absence of any one of these standards does not necessarily preclude a relationship between exposure and outcome, but may imply that further information is needed.

(4) Epidemiological evidence is usually collected from groups of people when it is impossible or impractical to collect experimental evidence, but once a causal relationship has been identified, experimental studies may be developed to test this.

2 Methods of studying nutrition: nutritional epidemiology

Aims

(1) To introduce nutritional epidemiology methods and their application.

(2) To consider advantages and disadvantages of available methods.

The role of nutrition in health is based on information about food intakes and about health indicators (*exposure* and *outcome*). This is addressed by nutritional epidemiology techniques in groups of people.

Study design

- Design is dictated by the research question to be asked (Table 2.1).
- Appropriate measurements must be used.
- Must compare like with like (*internal validity*) and ensure that any findings can be inferred back to the population from which the sample studied was drawn (*external validity*).

Measurements relevant to nutritional epidemiology

Investigations of the relationship between exposure and outcome cannot usually measure the *exact* exposure, as this will have occurred at an unspecified point or period of time. Therefore indirect markers, which can give an indication of the *exposure*, are used. Some of the same markers may also be indicative of *outcome*. Those most commonly used in nutritional studies are:

- food intake;
- biomarkers/clinical indicators;

- anthropometry.

Further, as diet-related behaviour does not exist in isolation, but is affected by *socio-demographic and cultural factors*, these may also need to be included in studies.

Assessment of food intake

This can be performed at group or individual level, depending on the nature of the study (Table 2.2).

Individual food intake measurement is the most common tool used in nutritional epidemiology (Table 2.3).

Food intake measures can be flawed: under-reporting can occur in all methods, as subjects fail to record, or alter their eating habits. This may account for up to 25% of intake; fat- and carbohydrate-rich foods are most likely to be under-reported. If energy intake falls below $1.2 \times$ the calculated BMR for an individual, it is highly likely to be under-reported.

Biomarkers

These include assessment of levels of nutrients or their derived products, such as enzymes (Table 2.4). Biomarkers may be influenced by hormone levels and activity of transport proteins, making it difficult to extrapolate to nutrient intake for some nutrients. Individual inherited differences in genes (polymorphisms) affect responses of markers both to nutrients and to lifestyle factors. New biomarkers related to molecular-level activities of nutrients or harmful agents are being developed.

Table 2.1 Examples of study designs used in nutritional epidemiology.

Type of study	Key features	Comment
Ecological study	Compare different areas, possibly over time Measure exposure to a factor (nutrient intake), against the prevalence rate of the disease (outcome)	Aggregated values may mask considerable individual differences
Cross-sectional design (prevalence studies)	Measure exposure and outcome at a point in time, in a population If repeated, can be used to monitor trends	Can make no statement that the exposure predated the outcome
Cohort study	Sample (cohort) studied at baseline and followed up to monitor new disease in those exposed/not exposed to the factor studied Relative risk (RR) is the incidence of disease in the exposed group compared to the unexposed group Can be used to study multiple outcomes and complex dietary patterns	Need very large numbers of subjects: expensive and resource demanding A retrospective cohort study can be performed if data of sufficient quality are available from a time in the past
Case-control studies	Data about exposure to the factor(s) being studied collected from people who have the outcome/disease and a matched sample without the disease	Recall of past diet is often poor, but particularly appropriate for diseases that are relatively uncommon in a population
Clinical trials (randomised controlled trials – RCTs)	Considered to be the 'gold standard' method Subjects randomly assigned to 'treatment' or 'control' group, with outcomes measured after some time	The challenge is to modify dietary intakes in such a way that only one factor is altered Ethical issues need to be considered in any design
Community trials	Intervention is made within a community, e.g. town, workplace, school Results compared between units in an experimental design	Can be useful for assessing the effectiveness of interventions over time

Table 2.2 Overview of methods of assessment of food intake.

Population sample studied	Method/source of data collected	Key features
National	Food balance sheets showing food produced/imported and food lost/exported	Gives a snapshot of food/nutrient availability; possibly per head of population No information about distribution of food
Household	Food inventory within a household; purchases and other incoming food recorded, usually over one week Food consumed outside the home may also be recorded	Distribution within household is not taken into account Food wastage not recorded Can be used for comparisons, e.g. socioeconomic, regional
Institution	Records food delivered to client group, using catering records and the number of meals served	May not record wastage; may assume equal distribution No record of additional food from outside
Individual	Prospective and retrospective methods available (see Table 2.3)	Choice of method depends on data required

Clinical indicators provide valuable information about the state of health of the study population. Measures used can include:
- blood pressure;
- plasma cholesterol levels;
- presence and function of teeth;
- presence of disease (infection, diabetes, cancer, bowel diseases);
- muscle function, grip strength.

Anthropometry

Specific measurements of body size and changes in proportions are important indicators of nutritional state. These include:
- Weight and height – used to calculate body mass index in adults (W/H^2), and as indicators of wasting and stunting in children.
- Circumferences: mid-arm muscle (MAMC) can indicate undernutrition in children; waist:hip ratio (WHR) is an indicator of central adiposity in adults.
- Skinfold thickness – is a measure of subcutaneous adipose tissue, and if measured at the appropriate sites (mid-biceps, mid-triceps,

Table 2.3 Examples of methods available for individual food intake assessment.

Method	Benefit/drawbacks
Prospective studies	
Weighed inventory	Should record all food eaten Time consuming, requires commitment and literacy/numeracy
Food diary with household measures (or photographs)	More flexible Less quantitatively accurate
Food checklist	Quick to use Limited by foods listed, lacks quantification
Retrospective studies	
24-hour recall or diet history	Information about recent intakes Requires stable dietary pattern, awareness of food intake and memory
Food frequency questionnaire	Can establish dietary patterns Requires awareness of quality and quantity of food intake

Table 2.4 Some examples of biomarkers used in nutritional epidemiology.

Short-term marker of intake (days)	Medium-term marker (weeks)	Long-term marker (months)
Vitamin C in urine, white blood cells (WBCs) and plasma Nitrogen in urine Potassium and sodium in urine Methane in breath (NSP intake) Plasma carotenoid Serum vitamin K	Haemoglobin in red blood cells (RBCs), reflects iron intakes Glutathione peroxidase in RBCs, dependent on selenium intake Doubly-labelled water for energy expenditure	Retinol in liver Selenium in toenails Circulating vitamin D Fatty acid profile of adipose tissue

subscapular and suprailiac) can be used to calculate percent body fat.

Almost all aspects of the study of nutrition have potential drawbacks. Some can be eliminated with careful planning and design of studies, and where possible with repeated measures. In attempting to link *exposure* to a causative (or preventive) factor, and a health (or disease) *outcome*, the multifactorial nature of relationships needs to be considered to prevent inappropriate conclusions being made.

3 Nutritional assessment of individuals

Aims

(1) To examine ways of obtaining information about the nutritional status of individuals.

(2) To explore the uses and limitations of such information.

The techniques used in nutritional epidemiology (see Chapter 2) are also suitable for assessment of individuals.

Food intakes

In assessing individual food intakes, a compromise often occurs between an accurate assessment and one that represents normal food intakes (Table 3.1).

Nutrient intakes are calculated using food composition tables. Estimation of portion sizes and allowance for wastage also needs to be considered.

Anthropometry

Height and weight are the most commonly used measures, as the equipment needed is relatively simple and widely available. Weighing scales, stadiometers and any tapes for surrogate height measures should be regularly calibrated.

In children, growth charts are available (e.g. UK Child Growth Foundation, WHO) to plot serial measurement of height/length,

weight and also head circumference during growth and development. Growth should follow a centile, and substantial drift from this needs to be investigated.

Assessment of undernutrition, and its treatment, can be made on the basis of weight and height measurements (Table 3.2).

In adults, height and weight are combined as Body Mass Index (BMI), calculated by dividing weight (kilograms) by height^2 (metres).

BMI is used in international comparisons, but it does have shortcomings:

- the association of excessive weight with fat deposits may not apply in muscular individuals;
- in older subjects, loss of height may give spurious results.

WHO has defined a number of BMI ranges; these represent risk of associated disease (Table 3.3). (For some population groups, such as South Asians, health risks may increase at lower levels of BMI, with a desirable range from 19–23, and obesity starting at >27.5.)

Problems in measuring weight and height may arise in individuals who are:

Bed or chair bound

Severely overweight

Unable to stand up vertically (or lie flat)

Surrogate measures of height are available:

Knee height/lower leg length, ulnar length or demispan may be used with appropriate equations (although results for height may vary between these measures, they are adequate for BMI assessment).

Table 3.2 Internationally used standards for assessment of undernutrition.

Measurement	Implication
Children	
Weight for age, <2 standard deviations (SD) (or 2Z scores) below reference	Underweight: insufficient food intake currently
Height for age, <2 SD (or 2Z scores) below reference	Stunting: chronic undernutrition, affecting linear growth
Weight for height, <2 SD (or 2Z scores) below reference	Wasting: acute growth disturbance, change in body proportions
Adults	
BMI <18.5 kg/m^2	Chronic energy deficiency due to poor food intake or chronic disease
BMI <17.0 kg/m^2	Reduced physical capacity likely to increase susceptibility to illness

---

Table 3.1 Type of information obtained by food intake assessment methods.

Method of assessment	Information provided	Uses/limitations
Duplicate diets	Accurate measure of what has been eaten	May not be typical diet of subject; used in metabolic studies. Expensive
Food record (weighed, household measures, food photographs, food models)	Current food intake in 'free living' individual; portion size information varies with method	Gives an indication of nutrient intake Often under-reported, food habits altered Affected by seasonality
Food frequency questionnaire	Typical food intake over a period of time; may be focused on particular foods of interest relevant to the study	Can establish dietary pattern, especially for food groups present/absent from the diet Reliant on memory and accurate assessment of frequencies
24-hour recall and diet history	Recent food intake or typical food intake pattern, obtained by direct questioning	May not capture a normal day Diet history requires skilled interviewer and time Can indicate deficiencies in the diet, and correlate with other nutritional assessments

Table 3.3 Classification of body fatness, based on BMI (WHO).

Category	BMI range (kg/m^2)
Normal weight	18.5–24.9
Overweight	25–29.9
Obesity – class 1	30–34.9
Obesity – class 2	35–39.9
Obesity – class 3 (morbid obesity)	>40.0

Circumferences

Waist circumference, midway between the lower rib margin and the iliac crest, taken at the end of expiration, reflects visceral adiposity, and is sensitive to weight changes. Based on waist circumference, 'action levels' have been defined, related to level of risk to health (Table 3.4).

If **hip circumference** is also measured at the largest part of the buttocks, the ratio of waist to hip circumference (WHR) can indicate the distribution of body fat between central and peripheral regions. A ratio above 0.8 in women and 0.9 in men is taken as a measure of abdominal obesity; increasing values indicate higher levels of risk.

Mid-arm circumference (MAC) is a measure of the circumference at the midpoint of the upper arm, which is used, together with measurement of subcutaneous body fat (by skinfold thickness at the mid-triceps), to assess muscle circumference (mid-arm muscle circumference MAMC), and therefore indicate any wasting.

Body composition

The body is traditionally viewed as being made up of several compartments:
- fat mass;
- fat-free mass (protein and mineral);
- total body water.

Skinfold calipers are used at specific sites in the body (mid-biceps, mid-triceps, subscapular and suprailiac) to assess the thickness of the subcutaneous layer of fat, which represents the major proportion of total body fat. By inputting the measurements into a prediction equation, the percentage of body fat can be calculated.

Table 3.4 Action levels for weight loss, based on waist circumference.

Action level	Waist circumference – women	Waist circumference – men
Normal	<80 cm	<94 cm
Level 1 – no further weight gain	80–88 cm	94–102 cm
Level 2 – high risk, needs medical advice	>88 cm	>102 cm

Other methods for measuring body composition

Densitometry – subjects are weighed in air and immersed in water; appropriate equations are used to calculate body fat from the difference in weights. *Air displacement plethysmography* removes the need to be submerged in water.

Imaging techniques – use *computed tomography* or *magnetic resonance imaging*, to visualise discrete deposits of body fat, especially in the visceral region. *Dual energy X-ray examination* (DEXA) can also be used to predict visceral fat deposits.

Bioelectrical impedance analysis (BIA) – measures the resistance (or impedance) to a small electric current passed through electrodes attached to the hands and feet. Resistance is related to the level of total body water and fat-free mass, which is inversely related to fat mass. Although widely used, the technique is subject to error related to food intake, level of hydration and environmental temperature.

Dilution techniques – body water can be estimated from the concentration of radioactive isotopes injected into the body.

Urinary excretion of metabolites – such as creatinine and nitrogen indicates turnover of body protein and is an indicator of the fat-free mass.

Clinical indicators and biomarkers

A wide range of physical, biochemical and haematological assessments can be used in individuals. In the clinical setting, a number of these are part of the screening and assessment of individuals for nutritional support.

Screening is generally performed with a quick and simple tool, which can be used by a trained member of the nursing or other staff, either in the hospital or other settings. Key points assessed are generally:
- Current body mass index.
- Weight loss (unintentional changes over the recent past).
- Ability to consume food – likelihood of future weight loss.

The *Malnutrition Universal Screening Tool* (MUST) is a validated tool, widely used in the UK for nutritional screening. On the basis of the score, a patient may be ranked from low to high risk, and can then be referred for a more in-depth nutritional assessment, by a dietitian or a member of the nutrition support team.

Summary

Nutritional assessment of individuals includes a number of approaches. Describing and assessing the nutritional intake can indicate where potential problems may exist and what intervention may be needed.

Inadequate nutritional intakes: causes

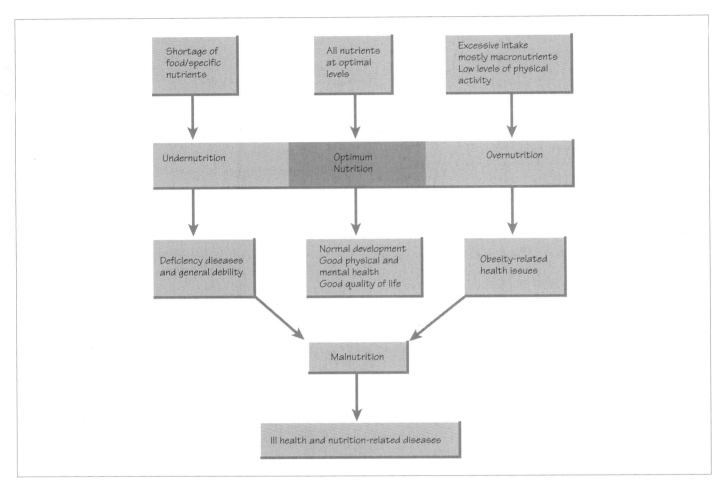

Fig. 4.1 Spectrum of nutrional adequacy.

Aims

(1) To consider how environmental factors may contribute to inadequate intakes.

(2) To recognise the extent of the problem of inadequate nutrition.

Inadequate intakes of specific nutrients and *excessive or unbalanced* intakes can both result in ill health (morbidity) and possibly death (mortality). The transition between these intake levels is difficult to define, so that nutritional adequacy is best viewed as a spectrum, rather than having fixed boundaries (Figure 4.1).

Causes of inadequate nutrition and associated disease

Who is at risk?

Individuals who live in countries with poor food security, or who themselves are food insecure, are at risk of undernutrition, which can manifest as hunger (chronic or seasonal), nutrient deficiencies or periods of starvation/famine.

Contributory factors

Disease prevalence is affected only in part by advances in medical practice and treatment. There are many *environmental* forces that have a much greater impact, as they affect all aspects of people's lives. Some examples are given in Table 4.1.

What actual impact these forces have on any single individual will ultimately be determined by the *personal choices* they make (or are able to make) as well as their individual *genetic susceptibility* to the effects of the environmental factors.

This *individual level of response* means that the effects of undernutrition may not be seen equally within a household, community or region.

Food supplies may be inadequate in quantity as well as quality so that inadequate energy intakes are likely to be accompanied by low intakes of other nutrients.

In some diets, nutrients may appear to be present, but are unavailable as a result of:

• binding to other components of the food (inactive form in the

Table 4.1 Potential impact of environmental factors on health outcomes.

Environmental factor	Consequence with potential impact on nutrition and health
Globalisation of crop production, trade and food supplies	Changes to food availability and dietary patterns in communities
Political and legislative measures	Policies on: health, education, agriculture and land ownership, import/export policies, employment, social/welfare policies, transport (food supplies, access to markets)
Socioeconomic status of groups within population	Access (physical and financial) to safe food of suitable nutritional quality Impact of status on living environment
Health-care provision	Access to appropriate health care at all life stages (e.g. immunisation, antenatal care, information on infant/child feeding practices, early recognition of disease)
Clean water and sanitation	Less infectious diseases and environmental contamination; reduced nutritional needs to fight infections
Education	Awareness of the importance of diet and health care, lifestyle habits Better food production techniques by farmers
Status of women	Women generally integrate health measures within a family; higher status allows women to be involved in decision-making

food, inactivated by food preparation methods, presence of phytate, dietary fibre);

• inhibition/promotion by other dietary factors eaten concurrently (e.g. factors affecting pH in the intestine);

• competition by parasitic infestation within the gut;

• poor utilisation, e.g. lack of carriers for absorption or transport in the blood, due to malnutrition;

• treatment with drugs preventing utilization.

Magnitude of the problem

It is difficult to obtain accurate information about the extent of undernutrition, because data are not collected routinely or are affected by sudden crises (war, environmental disasters) and the growing burden of disease such as HIV, AIDS and tuberculosis (TB) contributing to undernutrition.

Despite a theoretically adequate global food supply, the Food and Agriculture Organization (FAO) of the United Nations estimates that there are approximately 800 million undernourished people in the world, with the majority of these in the developing countries of the world, but also some 11 million in the developed countries. There have been reductions in the overall numbers in the last 20 years, but these vary between countries, with greatest progress in South America and parts of South-East Asia, and least progress in Africa.

In developed countries, inadequate intakes may be found in groups including:

• large families on low incomes;

• marginalised groups in society (e.g. minority ethnic groups, refugees, asylum seekers);

• the homeless;

• people with addictions (e.g. to drugs, alcohol);

• those in need of care who do not receive it (e.g. people with disabilities).

The consequences of inadequate nutrition will vary, and are discussed in Chapter 5.

5 Inadequate nutritional intakes: consequences

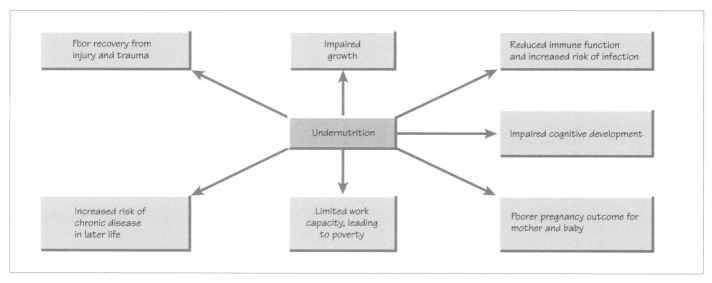

Fig. 5.1 Physiological and functional consequences of undernutrition.

Aims

(1) To consider the consequences of inadequate intake of macro-nutrients and micronutrients.

Inadequate intakes of macronutrients will most obviously be reflected in disturbed growth in children and body weight changes in adults.

Assessment

Anthropometric tools are used to assess the effects of under-nutrition (see Chapter 3). Measurements made in children, who are most dependent on their care-givers and therefore vulnerable, usually reflect the nutritional state of a community. Assessment of adolescents has been neglected in the past, due to the difficulty of relating measurements to reference standards during puberty. Undernutrition in the elderly is poorly reported, but is believed to be widespread, as this age group becomes increasingly dependent for food on more able-bodied members of their communities, as well as having a greater risk of disease, which can compromise nutritional status.

The *consequences* of undernutrition can manifest both in the short and long term, and may have intergenerational effects, through poor pregnancy outcome and low birth weight. These are summarised in Figure 5.1.

Specific manifestations of undernutrition
Macronutrient inadequacies

Protein-energy malnutrition, which reflects serious undernutrition, manifests as marasmus, kwashiorkor and a mixed picture of maras-mic kwashiorkor. The exact form of the condition depends on feeding patterns (Table 5.1).

Micronutrient inadequacies

Worldwide, deficiencies of iron, vitamin A and iodine affect the greatest numbers of people. However, several other micronutrients are now known to be widely deficient in populations and contribute to morbidity (Table 5.2).

Several other micronutrients may become deficient when diets lack specific food groups. These include:
- vitamin B_{12}, when vegan diets are consumed;
- calcium, when dairy products are excluded from the diet;
- riboflavin, when diets are low in green vegetables and dairy products.

Ensuring a balanced diet, containing appropriate amounts of foods from all major food groups (see Chapter 8), increases the chance of achieving adequate nutrition. Dietary variety helps to ensure an adequate diet, but may not always be possible if food supplies are limited.

Table 5.1 Conditions associated with a lack of macronutrients.

Condition	Diagnostic signs
Marasmus	Extreme wasting of fat stores and atrophy of visceral tissues; attributed to a severe lack of dietary energy Alert, but minimal physical activity undertaken Normal, but shrivelled skin Very susceptible to infection
Kwashiorkor	Oedema affecting face, limbs and abdomen, also enlarged liver Irritable, lethargic and anorexic Skin often cracked and ulcerated, hair colour changes Attributed to low protein intake, associated with excessive free radical damage to liver, with insufficient antioxidants
Marasmic kwashiorkor	Severe muscle wasting together with oedema Prognosis poor

Table 5.2 Conditions associated with a lack of micronutrients.

Nutrient	Numbers affected/causes	Consequences for health
Iron	About 5 billion people worldwide; mainly women and children Low iron intake or blood loss due to parasitic and malarial infections	Anaemia; affects cognitive development and behaviour in children, immune function, pregnancy outcome, work capacity
Vitamin A	Up to 250 million children with subclinical vitamin A deficiency (VAD); up to 500 000 become blind each year. Pregnant women also affected, transmits to next generation Low intake of preformed sources of vitamin A and low absorption rates of precursor carotenoids	In the eye: damage to cornea, leading to ulceration and blindness; loss of night vision Impaired resistance to infection, increased mortality Affects fetal development, physical growth, haemopoiesis, spermatogenesis
Iodine	Over 16 million children born with cretinism; up to 50 million affected with poor cognitive development Low levels in soils; goitrogens interfering with utilisation from the diet Low selenium levels may exacerbate low iodine intakes	Poor mental development in infants born to deficient mothers Stillbirths
Zinc	Up to 2 billion people Low dietary intake, high levels of absorption inhibitors	Increased risk of infection, reduced resistance Prematurity in infants, growth failure throughout childhood
Vitamin D	Numbers unknown; lack of exposure to sunlight, poor dietary intake, high levels of binding factors (e.g. phytate) in diet	Poor bone development in childhood and loss of bone minerals from mature bones

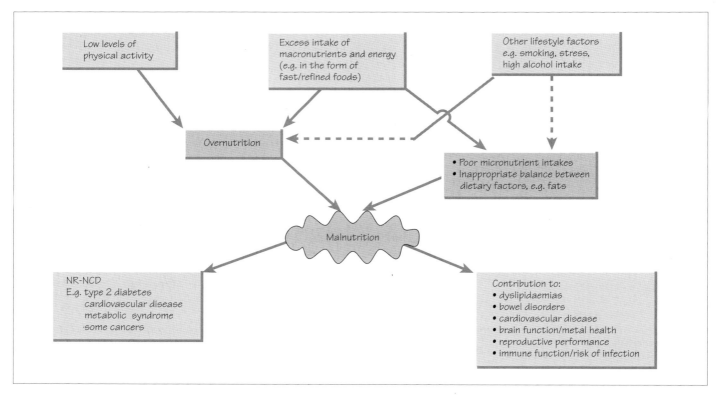

Fig. 6.1 Pathways to malnutrition from overnutrition and unbalanced diets.

Aims

(1) To recognise that overnutrition and unbalanced diets can result in malnutrition.

(2) To identify the dietary factors most likely to be associated with overnutrition and unbalanced diets.

Overnutrition and unbalanced diets can lead to increased morbidity and mortality from *nutrition-related non-communicable diseases* (NR-NCDs). These are generally multifactorial in origin, and the relationship between nutrition and diseases is less clear cut than in the case of specific deficiency diseases.

Traditionally associated with Western society, and previously termed 'diseases of affluence', these diseases now coexist in societies where substantial proportions of the population still suffer from undernutrition, imposing a double burden on health provision (Table 6.1).

Development of overnutrition and NR-NCDs

NR-NCDs occur in societies that have undergone a number of transitions, including:

• improvements in health care and infection control, thereby increasing life span;

• greater productivity;

• opportunities to improve living standards and thereby acquire more food;

Table 6.1 Prevalence of NR-NCDs.

	Worldwide	Developing countries	Industrialised/higher income economies
Deaths currently attributable to NR-NCDs	60%	40%	75%
Projected deaths due to NR-NCDs by 2020	73%	Up to 77% of deaths	Increases continuing in Eastern Europe and Middle Eastern countries

• increased industrialisation and urbanisation, resulting in reduced workloads (energy expenditure);

• globalisation leading to introduced foods with higher energy densities, increasing energy consumption.

In the West, where such changes occurred in the twentieth century, a further transition is now occurring with health promotion and education measures to enable individuals to actively work to reverse the consequences of these changes.

Both overnutrition and unbalanced diets result in manifestations of malnutrition with consequent ill health. These are summarised in Figure 6.1.

Dietary components and nutrients responsible for overnutrition and unbalanced diets

A number of dietary factors play a key role in the development of nutrition-related diseases. These are summarised in Table 6.2.

Fat

Many 'fast foods' or convenience products contain high levels of fat. A diet rich in fat is likely to lead to overconsumption of energy, and positive energy balance. Regulation of fat intake is poor, resulting in 'passive' overconsumption. Reducing the percentage fat in the diet is generally associated with weight loss.

Specific components of fat intake are also potentially associated with disease.
- Saturated fats are positively related to plasma cholesterol levels and risk of coronary heart disease.
- An appropriate ratio of saturated, monounsaturated and poly-unsaturated fats is important in terms of protection against coronary heart disease.
- A balance between *n*-3 and *n*-6 fatty acids is desirable for brain development, mental health, possibly coronary heart disease and inflammatory responses.

Sugar

Foods and drinks containing high levels of sugar have spread around the world as part of the globalisation of food supplies.
- High levels of sugar intake are mainly associated with dental caries, especially if the sugar is consumed in a sticky form and between rather than with meals.
- Consumption of soft drinks, containing 'hidden' sugar in solution, results in excessive energy consumption and may contribute to overweight in young people.
- Sugar *per se* is not a causative factor in overweight or type 2 diabetes. Diets high in sugar are often lower in fat and so are less obesogenic.

Complex carbohydrates

Generally these are more slowly digested and absorbed from the gastrointestinal tract and as such have a lower glycaemic effect and fewer metabolic consequences.

- Many foods rich in complex carbohydrates are also rich in dietary fibre; consumed within normal limits, fibre is beneficial in terms of weight control and bowel function.
- Excessive amounts can be detrimental, as they are very satiating and may result in an overall energy intake that does not meet requirements. Care is needed in people with small appetites, such as children and older adults.

Alcohol

- Alcohol can contribute to excessive energy intakes, when taken in addition to normal food consumption. However, not all studies show an association between large intakes of alcohol and weight gain.
- Alcohol intake may disrupt normal food intake, leading to under-nutrition or potentially malnutrition, with excessive energy, coupled with poor micronutrient intake resulting from a lack of dietary quality.

Antioxidant nutrients

This group, which is most commonly taken to mean vitamins C and E and the carotenoids, may be inadequate in diets that are rich in macronutrients, but have low dietary quality. Such diets are likely to contain low amounts of fruit and vegetables, despite an apparently adequate intake of energy.
- A large body of research implicates low antioxidant status in the development of NR-NCD, although supplementation trials with the individual antioxidants have not provided the expected beneficial results.

Nutritional supplements

There is potential for harm from excessive intakes of nutrients, usually in the form of supplements.
- There are physiological mechanisms regulating absorption, transport or excretion in the body that generally protect the system from potentially toxic levels of nutrients. These may fail in certain conditions, such as excessive alcohol intake, genetic disorders or renal disease affecting nutrient excretion.
- For many nutrients it is possible for excessive amounts to be taken into the body and eventually to cause harmful effects. These include some of the water-soluble vitamins (e.g. vitamins B_6, C and folate), fat-soluble vitamins (e.g. vitamins A and D) and many of the minerals (e.g. copper, iron, magnesium and selenium).
- For this reason, many countries, as well as the FAO/WHO, have established upper limits for safe intakes, which are intended for use with nutritional supplements, to safeguard consumers against excessive intakes.

Conclusion

Although the nutrition transition has brought benefits in terms of an end to hunger and undernutrition for *some* population groups, these have come at a price, of overweight and its comorbidities. Protective factors in traditional diets have been lost.

Within countries, and even within households, there are sub-groups who have benefitted with better nutrition, while others remain affected by hunger. This poses a major challenge for health provision and to health planners.

Table 6.2 Key dietary factors linked to overnutrition or unbalanced diets.

Overconsumed	Underconsumed
Fats, total levels; also saturated and possibly *n*-6 fatty acids	*n*-3 fatty acids, especially in relation to high intakes of *n*-6 fatty acids
Sources of refined carbohydrate, e.g. sugars, products with high glycaemic index	Complex carbohydrates, with low glycaemic index, e.g. whole plant foods
Alcoholic beverages	Antioxidant nutrients, present in foods of plant origin, such as fruit and vegetables
Salt (as sodium), particularly from processed foods	Potassium (e.g. from fruit and vegetables), which may counterbalance high sodium intakes
Nutritional supplements, not excreted from the body	

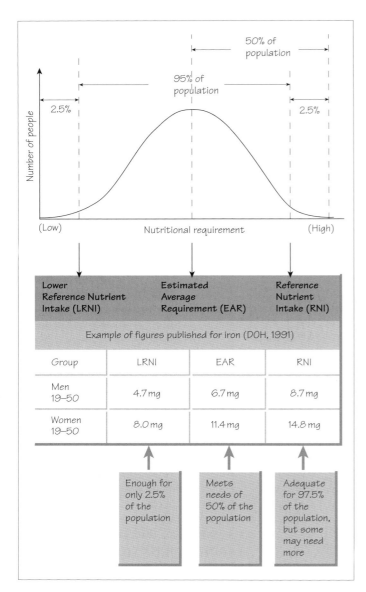

Fig. 7.1 Basis of dietary reference values.

Aims

(1) To define nutritional requirements.

(2) To explain the basis of dietary recommendations for energy and nutrients.

In defining an adequate diet, distinction should be made between the *physiological need* for essential nutrients and the *balance of foods to be eaten* to provide these.

• Information about the appropriate quantities of nutrients can be obtained from a study of nutritional requirements, which can lead to recommendations for dietary reference values and nutrient-based dietary goals, aimed at groups or populations.

• However, people do not eat food with the conscious awareness that they are consuming nutrients, and for practical purposes, any

definitions of an adequate diet must be expressed in terms of food-based guidelines, aimed at individuals. In order to do this, knowledge of the major nutrient groups provided by foods is required (this is considered in Chapter 8).

Nutritional requirements

A certain amount of every nutrient is used by the body every day. This amount must therefore be replaced, either from the diet or from body stores.

For some nutrients a daily intake is not crucial as the amount used is a small proportion of that available in the body. However, if the daily needs are provided from body stores over a period of time, then the stores gradually become depleted, the functional form of the nutrient becomes unavailable and eventually a clinical deficiency develops.

For other nutrients there is little or no storage, and therefore a regular intake is necessary. In general, it is therefore preferable to aim for a daily intake of all nutrients and so ensure a continued adequate provision.

A *requirement* is defined as the amount of a specific nutrient required by an individual to prevent clinical signs of deficiency. Two problems arise from this definition:

• the possibility that depletion of reserves to a level short of clinical deficiency may be harmful to health, or that amounts greater than the minimum may have a positively beneficial effect;

• quantifying requirements of nutrients for which there is no definable deficiency state.

Nevertheless, ascertaining nutrient requirements is necessary for guidance on adequate diets.

Dietary Reference Values (DRVs)

Requirements within a population group are generally assumed to be normally distributed (Figure 7.1).

It has become accepted that in order to translate these into recommendations for populations, and to cover the requirements of the majority, a value set at two standard deviations above the average requirement is used. By the nature of a normal distribution curve, this encompasses 97.5% of the population, and as such represents a value that is greater than the needs of the majority. In the UK this level is known as the Reference Nutrient Intake (RNI); in the European Union (EU) and USA the same level is termed the Recommended Dietary Allowance (RDA).

In addition, a value set at the average requirement minus two standard deviations is used as the least amount that might be adequate for all but 2.5% of the population. This is termed the Lower Reference Nutrient Intake (LRNI) in the UK.

For energy, the Estimated Average Requirement (EAR) is used; this can be applied to a group, some of whom will have needs lower than this and some higher than this. The mean intake for the group should equal the EAR if it is to be concluded that individual needs are being met.

For some nutrients, like fat, carbohydrate and dietary fibre, where specific deficiency states cannot be identified, requirements are more difficult to set. In the UK, needs for these nutrients are based on evidence relating to reducing the risk of chronic disease, where this is available. Values are expressed as a percentage of total energy intake that should be provided by different types of fat and carbohydrates.

For a small number of nutrients insufficient information is available to set requirements and RNI, so a 'safe intake' (UK) or Adequate Intake (USA) is used to give a general target figure.

All of these figures, as currently used in the UK, are set out in the COMA (Committee on Medical Aspects of Food Policy) Report 41 (*Dietary Reference Values for Food Energy and Nutrients for the United Kingdom*), first published by the Department of Health in 1991. Figures are given for different age groups, and in separate categories for males and females (see Appendix 3).

Similar sets of figures are published in other countries, as well as by the EU and the FAO/WHO, and are reviewed on a regular basis. These figures often exhibit some diversity, reflecting the thinking of the committees involved in their preparation.

For **food labelling**, the UK uses EU figures for RDAs, which are based on the values for an adult male, aged 19–50 (except for iron, which is based on the higher, female figure). This is also the case in the USA, where the higher figure of male or female values for adults under the age of 50 years, is used in food labelling.

Guideline Daily Amounts (GDA) have recently been introduced in the UK as a means of simplifying the concept of recommended amounts. A single figure for a GDA is used, averaging recommendations for males and females. This allows the food label to show the contribution made by an average serving to the daily needs. An example is shown in Table 7.1.

Conclusion

Values for nutritional requirements, expressed in the form of dietary recommendations or reference values for nutrients, provide the basis for dietary advice. However, to be usable these values need to be expressed in terms of foods. This is considered in Chapter 8.

Table 7.1 Example of a food label (from a breakfast cereal) showing Guideline Daily Amounts.

Nutrient[a]	Guideline Daily Amount[b]	Each serving, with milk[c]	Percentage of Guideline Daily Amount[d]
Calories	2000 kcal	225 kcal	11
Sugar	90 g	15.7 g	17
Fat	70 g	2.7 g	4
Saturated fat	20 g	1.5 g	8

[a]Nutrients selected reflect those seen as key to 'healthy eating'.

[b]Values calculated from Dietary Reference Values, as an average of adult male and female values. A note on the label may suggest that men may need slightly more and women and young people may need slightly less than this, but it is not quantified.

[c]Based on a 50-g serving of the cereal product, with 125 mL of semi-skimmed milk. Full fat milk would increase the fat contents.

[d]Allows consumers to see at a glance how much of their daily needs have been met.

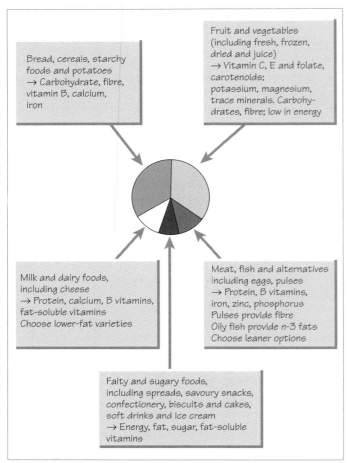

Bread, cereals, starchy foods and potatoes
→ Carbohydrate, fibre, vitamin B, calcium, iron

Fruit and vegetables (including fresh, frozen, dried and juice)
→ Vitamin C, E and folate, carotenoids; potassium, magnesium, trace minerals. Carbohydrates, fibre; low in energy

Milk and dairy foods, including cheese
→ Protein, calcium, B vitamins, fat-soluble vitamins
Choose lower-fat varieties

Meat, fish and alternatives including eggs, pulses
→ Protein, B vitamins, iron, zinc, phosphorus
Pulses provide fibre
Oily fish provide n-3 fats
Choose leaner options

Fatty and sugary foods, including spreads, savoury snacks, confectionery, biscuits and cakes, soft drinks and ice cream
→ Energy, fat, sugar, fat-soluble vitamins

Fig. 8.1 Diagrammatic representation of the Plate Model.

Aims

(1) To describe 'healthy eating'.

(2) To show how dietary recommendations can be used in a variety of ways to produce guidelines for an adequate diet.

It can be anticipated that an *adequate diet* will be one that:

- contains all of the nutrients listed in the DRV tables, in amounts that meet the RNI, for the particular age and sex of the individual;
- supports health, and allows the fulfilment of all the work and leisure activities desired by an individual;
- provides sufficient reserve to protect the individual from nutritional deficiency during periods of poor food intake, for example during short periods of illness;
- offers some protection against disease.

These points could be said to encompass the principles of 'healthy eating', and by implication, diets that do not achieve the above goals might be considered 'unhealthy'. However, without the necessary information about nutrient contents of foods, found in food composition tables, this is not something that can be readily checked by an individual consumer.

Advice on healthy eating can be formulated in fairly general terms, such as those produced by the Food Standards Agency in the UK:
- Base your meals on starchy foods.
- Eat lots of fruit and veg.
- Eat more fish – including a portion of oily fish each week.
- Cut down on saturated fat and sugar.
- Try to eat less salt – no more than 6 g a day for adults.
- Get active and try to be a healthy weight.
- Drink plenty of water.
- Don't skip breakfast.

Practical suggestions for 'healthy eating' can be explained to consumers, with advice on implementation. They can also form the basis for more detailed advice, such as that produced in the form of food-based guidelines.

A balanced diet

The concept of the '*balanced diet*' has been developed on the basis of the nutritional composition of related foods, which can be classified into groups. By constructing diets containing appropriate amounts of these food groups, relative to one another, it is possible to arrive at a diet that contains foods and therefore nutrients that are 'balanced'.

This has now been linked to advice on healthy eating in a variety of *food planning guides,* such as the 'pyramid' (as used in the USA, Asia and the Mediterranean) or 'plate' (as used in the UK) models. In general these all recommend that the diet is principally made up of plant foods – grains, pulses, fruit and vegetables rather than animal sources.

The Plate Model (Balance of Good Health)

According to the UK's Plate Model, the cereals and starchy foods group and fruit and vegetables group should each comprise one third of the diet. The remaining third should predominantly be composed of meat, fish and alternatives (12%) and dairy products (15%), with only a small proportion of the diet coming from foods rich in fat and sugar (8%) (Figure 8.1).

Not every meal should necessarily be made up of all these components, but over the course of a day, the food eaten should achieve this balance, to ensure a healthy diet. By aiming for this balance of foods, a balanced intake of nutrients should follow.

Some additional advice has evolved from the original concept of the Plate Model, such as the promotion of 'five a day' for fruit and vegetables, or 'three a day' for the dairy products group. This may make it easier for some people to monitor their intake, but can also seem an unachievable target and be discouraging.

It should be remembered that the Plate Model, like the other pictorial representations used in various countries, is simply a guide,

Applying the 'Plate Model'

Although the principle of the Plate Model is straightforward, its application sometimes causes problems. The main questions asked by consumers are:

- Which groups do composite dishes count towards (e.g. meat and vegetable mixtures, pizzas)?
- How big is a portion?
- What about alcohol?
- Does it apply to the very young, and old, people with small appetites, or on special diets?
- Is it suitable for people in the UK from different cultures. This has been addressed by the development of modified versions of the Plate Model that include foods traditional to these groups.

and provides an overview of the relative proportions of the diet – it is not meant to be prescriptive, as there are very many different ways of achieving a balanced diet.

The *key objective is to consume a mixture of foods*, and include as much variety as possible.

No foods are specifically excluded, and none are essential – there is no implicit labelling of 'good' and 'bad' foods. However, some foods should be eaten in greater amounts, and perhaps be included at all meals, and some should be eaten only occasionally, and perhaps seen as occasional 'treats', rather than an everyday item.

'Traffic light' labelling

Advances in the way foods are labelled are being developed in the UK to provide a further tool to help consumers choose foods that can contribute to a balanced diet. Based on a target level of intake for particular nutrients, foods may be labelled with a series of traffic light symbols for specific nutrients: green, amber and red to provide a guide to foods that can be eaten freely without compromising dietary quality and those whose intake should be limited. This is an area of debate, as some foods may be 'green' for one nutrient, but 'red' for another.

Conclusion

By using food-based dietary guidelines and pictorial representations of a balanced diet, together with additional information on food labels, it is intended that consumers achieve an adequate and healthy diet. In this way, despite not necessarily being aware of nutritional requirement figures, the consumer will actually fulfil these from the food eaten.

9 Food choice: internal and external factors

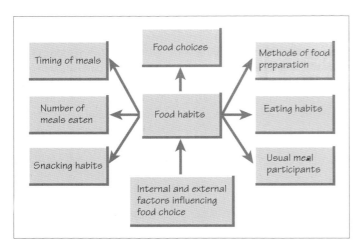

Fig. 9.1 Main components of food habits within group/culture.

Aims
(1) To describe the internal factors that influence an individual's food choice.
(2) To identify the external factors that shape an individual's food choice.

In order to achieve an intake of nutrients that meets physiological requirements, and provides for optimal health, it is necessary to make an *appropriate selection of foods*. Many factors determine this selection – they can be categorised as ones relating to:
• the individual consumer (internal factors);
• the cultural and social context (external factors);
• the food itself (considered in Chapter 10).
Understanding these factors and their impact on consumer choices is critical in any initiative that attempts to change food intakes. The relationship between these factors is complex, and individuals are often unconscious of the influences, making it a difficult area for study.

Food habits
Food choices comprise one part of the wider attribute of *food habits*, which are the typical behaviours of a group of people in relation to food.

They are seen to provide an important signal of group identity. In addition to the foods chosen, food habits will also determine eating times and numbers of meals, food preparation methods and meal participants, portion sizes and ways of eating. Food habits are the product of environmental influences on a culture, and as such are generally slow to change (Figure 9.1).

Internal factors determining food choices
Physiological and psychological factors underpin the drive to eat. Table 9.1 summarises the main internal factors that play a role in determining food choice.

All of the factors listed in Table 9.1 can be classified as internal biological responses. Psychological influences may modify or override the physiological need for food; examples of this include binge eating, or refusal to eat as a result of depression.

Internal factors cannot be separated from the external environment that will have shaped the setting in which these responses have developed. For example, dietary restraint is likely to have developed as a response to a cultural norm for slimness in women; perceptions and preferences for foods may then be shaped by this norm, and become a behaviour influencing food choice.

Control over food choice
It is important to recognise the existence of internal factors in food choice, and allow individuals control over their food choice. Loss of control can lead to loss of appetite; which may be a problem in institutions where menus are centrally determined. Subjects who are prescribed modified diets may also experience a loss of control with consequently poor adherence to the diet.

Table 9.1 Summary of the main physiological and psychological factors believed to have a role in the internal control of food choice.

Factor	Expression	Comments
Physiological factors		
Hunger	Need to eat	Often determined by habit
Satiation/satiety	Stops food intake/prevents subsequent eating	May be over-ridden if presented with a variety of foods
Psychological factors		
Appetite	Desire for specific foods, based on experience	Not thought to be linked to nutritional need
Aversion	Avoidance of specific foods, from (perceived) experience	May severely restrict food choices
Preference	Established by frequency of exposure and early learning. May also be linked to genetic differences in taste sensitivities	Sets specific taste thresholds, e.g. to sugar, salt; also resistance to new tastes (neophobia). Reinforced by positive outcomes (e.g. increased alertness)
Emotions (mood, stress)	Specific foods associated with positive or negative emotions	May lead to comfort eating, or food refusal as a weapon
Personality traits	Sensitivity to external and internal cues affecting food intake	May be important in belief about ability to control body weight

External factors

These are determined by the social and cultural context, and inevitably also affect both development and persistence of internal factors, as well as the food available.

Culture

Culture is a major determinant of food choice; it confers and reinforces identity and belonging, and underlines differences from other cultures. Cultural influences may be overt (staple food, most popular dish) or subtle (seasonings used, method of cooking). The finding that migrants maintain cultural identity by retaining food choices has been reported in many studies.

Culture defines what is acceptable as food, and may identify subgroups for whom certain foods are acceptable. For example, not all food is considered appropriate for children or in pregnancy (e.g. alcoholic drinks).

Religion

Religion frequently determines the broad context of food choice, with a number of world religions laying down rules about what is permitted, and when it may or may not be eaten. Prohibitions exist on different types of meat, meat in general and methods of slaughter; cooking methods and food combinations are also governed by rules. Rules may also cover periods of fasting, rituals and festivals. Followers of these religions experience constraint in food choice, but also gain a sense of identity.

Ethical decisions

The way food is produced may affect food choices. There are many concerns about rearing animals for food and environmentally damaging methods of agriculture. Supporters may alter their food choices to match their ethical principles, choosing organically produced food, becoming vegan or vegetarian.

Economic factors

For individuals within any cultural or religious group, access to food in terms of money or goods for exchange is a critical factor determining choice. More and greater variety of food can be obtained with higher economic status. Conversely, people in poverty or on a low income have limited opportunity to exercise alternative food choices. This may be the result of poor availability of food in their locality, inadequate money to buy food or a combination of both.

Social norms

The accepted behaviour within an individual's social circle in relation to food plays a strong influence on food choice. This is exerted through peer pressure and reinforces expectations about food. It may perpetuate food choices along gender lines, where some foods are perceived as more 'masculine' (red meat, beer), whereas others are more 'feminine' (salads, white wine). Social norms may also determine the status of foods – with some foods being perceived as more prestigious (often expensive) and therefore used to impress others, used on special occasions only, or never eaten as being 'not for the likes of me'.

Education/health awareness

This originates from the external environment and determines engagement with food and nutrition issues and the degree to which health issues influence food choice. Many barriers, including some of the other external influences discussed here, may exist that interfere with this process. The recognition of risk from an unhealthy diet, its relevance to the individual and the ability to act on this by food choices are key prerequisites.

Media and advertising

These provide information about some foods, usually those that have been processed or manufactured, and possibly less nutritionally desirable with higher levels of fat, salt and sugar. Exposure to advertising for food items increases awareness of and demand for the product. Children from lower income households who watch most television have the highest intake of advertised foods.

Conclusion

Social and cultural factors have a great influence on food choice, even when consumers are not conscious of this. These modify or over-ride physiological and psychological factors, and can have both positive and negative consequences on total food intake.

Food choice: the food environment

Aims

(1) To consider the classification of foods within diets.
(2) To show how the nature of the food influences food choice.

The globalisation of food has resulted in many changes in the diets of populations around the world. This changing food environment has an inevitable effect on food choices, as traditional foods lose their predominance in the diet and are replaced by more novel foods. Expectations about food choices also change as foods that were only seasonally available may now be obtained at other times of the year.

Classification of foods

Traditionally diets have been described as composed of core, secondary and peripheral foods (Table 10.1). The knowledge of what constitutes a 'meal' has been transmitted through generations. New foods have been subsumed into this structure, as they have become available. Food choice therefore has been made on the basis of foods that when eaten together would constitute a meal, or were suitable as a snack.

The concept of a meal has also changed for some, with a pattern of smaller snacks being consumed during the day. Some snacks continue to fit into the patterns shown in Table 10.1: for example, a sandwich comprises bread (cereal) plus filling (secondary food); a packet of crisps is essentially a starchy food (potato), albeit with added fat. Others comprise just a secondary food, such as a piece of fruit, or a milk-based drink. However, other snacks, such as confectionery or soft drinks, are peripheral foods, often with low nutritional value.

Developments in food technology have created many new foods in recent years, which do not all fit into the traditional pattern of meals. For example, breakfast cereal bars are designed to be eaten on the way to work, and can be considered neither as a meal nor a snack. Meal replacement drinks, sold to encourage weight loss, do not fit into any of the above categories. Nutrients added to enrich certain products, for example, calcium added to orange juice, alter the nutritional 'identity' of such items. This creates difficulties for health educators in terms of advising on dietary changes.

The nature of the food available

For food choice to occur, the food itself must be available and palatable, and consumers must know about it. Food availability depends on consumers' access to shops and markets, which is variable. In some areas 'food deserts' with few or no shops have been described. There is also concern about how far food is transported, as consumers become more aware of the environmental costs of 'food miles'. Palatability is the ultimate determinant of food choice – consumers will refuse to buy, or will not buy again, foods that they find unpalatable. This creates a challenge for the food producer and food technologist, as well as for quality controllers to minimise spoilage and maintain safety of the product.

Table 10.1 Traditional classification of foods within diets.

Core foods	Secondary foods	Peripheral foods
Foods that tend to occur in the diet several times in the day – usually include the 'staple' food of the population group, e.g. cereal, starchy foods *Nutritionally*: generally a source of energy, carbohydrate, some protein, some minerals and vitamins	Foods that enhance the meal, by adding variety and extra colour/texture/flavour; not considered vital to have at every meal Often include sources of protein, e.g. meat, fish, dairy products, pulses, vegetables and fruit *Nutritionally*: a source of protein, additional minerals and vitamins	Foods that are not considered an essential part of the diet, but are pleasant to eat May be seen as a treat or extra item May also include foods only eaten at special occasions Include drinks, e.g. tea, coffee, wine *Nutritionally*: may be rich in fats and sugars

Table 10.2 Summary of the major factors associated with availability and palatability of foods.

	Factors involved	Comments
Availability of food	Physical/geographical factors in production Transport and marketing arrangements (for both the food and the consumer) Storage facilities	Large out-of-town shops may limit access for some consumers 24-hour shopping can increase availability Small convenience stores may not sell healthy items
Palatability	Appeal to the visual and olfactory senses is the key to initial selection Taste, flavour and texture (hedonic appeal) also determine palatability	Criteria of palatability vary with different foods Fat and sugar combinations often associated with high levels of hedonic appeal Advertisers have to overcome resistance to new, unknown flavours and textures

Aspects involved in availability and palatability are summarised in Table 10.2.

Food choice is an immensely complicated issue. Individual, social and cultural factors interact together with the food environment to influence individual behaviour. The food environment itself is the product of many commercial decisions, reflected in marketing strategies, pricing policies and advertising. The influences discussed in Chapters 9 and 10 are summarised in Table 10.3.

Table 10.3 Summary of influences on food choice.

Internal (individual) factors	External (social/cultural) factors	Nature of the food
Appetite	Culture	Availability
Aversion	Religion	Palatability
Preference	Ethical decisions	
Emotions	Economic factors	
Personality traits	Social norms	
Mood and stress	Education/health awareness	
	Media and advertising	

Changing food choices

Research on moving consumers towards healthier food choices has not been very systematic to date. It is very difficult to make a large change in food choice, monitor and measure this and study any health outcome. Thus tailored approaches are needed that address different groups in the population and particular aspects of food choice.

Specific strategies that are appropriate for the target group are proposed. These might include computer-based or SMS-text interventions for young people, supermarket-based interventions for women, sports club- or pub-based interventions for young men, and peer-led interventions for children, adolescents and ethnic minority groups.

The environment in which change is expected must be supportive and not conflict with the aims of the change process.

Only by integrating what is known about factors that influence food choice with proposed intervention methods can change be achieved.

11 Introduction to the nutrients

Aims

(1) To classify nutrients in various ways and show their main roles.

(2) To show that nutrients may interact to fulfil similar roles.

• Food is composed of a large variety of chemical substances.

• Some are recognised as *nutrients*, and nutrition science has identified their roles and the consequences of insufficient intakes.

• Many others are present, especially in foods of plant origin; these promote the plant's growth, protect it against predators, or contribute to its appearance or smell to attract animals that will spread its seeds. These substances (*phytochemicals*) are not recognised as nutrients but may be bioactive and have beneficial and harmful effects within humans.

Classification of nutrients

The major nutrients have traditionally been classified according to the amounts in which they are required, their chemical nature and their functions in the body. A principal distinction is between macronutrients and micronutrients.

(1) *Macronutrients* are required in large amounts by the body, usually measured in tens of grams.

(2) *Micronutrients* are substances required in very small amounts by the body, generally measured in milligrams or micrograms. Some classifications also include *ultratrace nutrients*, found in the diet in quantities less than 1 μg/g of dry diet; roles for many of these are unknown.

Water is an essential component of the diet, as an adequate intake of fluid is vital to sustain life.

Macronutrients

The macronutrients found in the diet are carbohydrates, fats and proteins.

• Carbohydrates and fats are the major *providers of energy*, although protein can also provide energy.

• They all have a *structural* role, the most important in this respect being proteins.

• All contain *carbon, hydrogen* and *oxygen*; in addition, proteins contain nitrogen and some contain sulphur.

Carbohydrates

These are saccharides, combined in various degrees of complexity to form the simple sugars, and larger units such as oligosaccharides and polysaccharides. Their main function is to act as a source of energy, in the form of glucose. Some resist digestion (termed 'nonglycaemic'), and comprise the non-starch polysaccharides (NSP), which are part of 'dietary fibre' and have a role in bowel function.

Fats

Fats comprise a diverse group of lipid-soluble substances, the majority being triglycerides or triacylglycerols (TAGs). Derived products such as phospholipids and sterols (most notably cholesterol) are included in this group.

TAGs are broken down to yield energy, and form the major energy reserve in the body, in adipose tissue. Specific fatty acids found in TAGs are important in cell membrane structure and function, and must be supplied in the diet. These are termed *essential fatty acids*.

Proteins

Proteins consist of chains of individual amino acids, combined to form a large variety of proteins. On digestion, individual amino acids are used for the synthesis of other amino acids and proteins required by the body, involving considerable recycling of the components.

There are eight 'essential amino acids' (more in children), which must be supplied by the diet. In addition, some may become 'conditionally' essential in particular situations of physiological stress. Only when there is no further need for amino acids are they broken down and used as a source of energy, and the nitrogen part excreted as urea.

Micronutrients

The micronutrients comprise the minerals and vitamins (Table 11.1).

Minerals

These are inorganic substances needed in small amounts, generally as part of the structure of other molecules (e.g. iron as part of hae-

---

Interactions

When food is eaten, possible interactions between the various nutrients and non-nutritional constituents can occur at all stages of the processing and metabolism of the food within the body. It is therefore unwise to study nutrients in isolation without considering some of the other factors that may influence their activity and how they may interact in whole body functioning.

Table 11.1 Classification of micronutrients by chemical properties.

Name	Main members of the group	Role(s)
Minerals	Calcium, phosphorus, sodium, potassium, iron, zinc, copper, magnesium, selenium	Structural role Cofactors for enzymes Acid–base balance
Water-soluble vitamins	B vitamin group; vitamin C	Metabolism; cell division; antioxidant; cofactors for enzymes Synthesis of neurotransmitters
Fat-soluble vitamins	Vitamins A, D, E, K	Structural, cell integrity Homeostasis Antioxidant role

moglobin), or as essential cofactors for the activity of enzymes (e.g. selenium in glutathione peroxidase).

Uptake of some minerals from the diet must be carefully regulated as there is limited excretion, and potential toxicity may result if large amounts accumulate in storage organs.

In addition some minerals compete with each other for absorption, so excessive intakes of one may hinder uptake of another (e.g. zinc and iron, or iron and calcium).

Vitamins

These share the common feature of being organic substances, required by the body in small amounts for its normal functioning.

The vitamins are subclassified, into water-soluble (vitamin C and B vitamins) and fat-soluble (vitamins A, D, E and K) groups.

It is now recognised that *vitamin D* is synthesised in the skin by the action of ultraviolet light on a precursor, and could strictly be termed a hormone rather than a vitamin. Further, *niacin* can be made in the body from the amino acid tryptophan, so a separate supply may not be needed if protein intakes are adequate. However, in both of these cases, there are situations where synthesis is insufficient, and so a dietary need remains.

Water

Water provides the basic medium in which all the body's reactions occur. An inadequate level of fluid intake will quickly compromise the metabolic functions of the body and disturb the homeostatic mechanisms that operate.

Alcohol is not considered to be a nutrient. However, when ingested it can provide energy, and some alcoholic beverages provide additional nutrients, albeit in small amounts.

Nutrient interactions

Many nutrients interact in functional roles (Table 11.2).
• At the genetic level, nutrients are involved in the transcription of genes, regulating the synthesis of proteins and enzymes.
• At the cellular level, nutrients are involved as cofactors in controlling and regulating metabolic reactions and releasing energy from other nutrients. They are regulated by hormones and other chemical messengers, such as cytokines, which are also influenced by the nutrient environment.

Table 11.2 Grouping of micronutrients by functional role in the body.

Function	Micronutrients involved
Blood and circulation, maintenance of homeostasis	Iron, vitamin B_{12}, folate Vitamin K and calcium Electrolytes: sodium and potassium
Cellular and whole body metabolism	Thiamin, riboflavin, niacin, pyridoxine Zinc, magnesium, biotin, pantothenic acid Iodine
Protective/defence mechanisms	Vitamin C, vitamin E, β-carotene, selenium
Structural	Calcium, vitamin D, vitamin K Vitamin A

• Immune and defence mechanisms function through release of free radicals, which must then be quenched by antioxidants, again supplied directly by the diet or indirectly as enzymes activated by dietary factors.

Key characteristics of nutrients
In studying the nutrients it is necessary to know:
• their structure and characteristics;
• which foods are major sources;
• how they are processed by the digestive tract, absorbed, transported and stored;
• in what form they are used, what determines their use, how they are mobilised and in what circumstances, how surplus or metabolic end products are excreted;
• what the physiological requirement for the nutrient is, and how this can be translated into a recommended level of intake;
• how the body responds to overconsumption and underconsumption;
• how long it takes to develop a deficiency syndrome and what are the characteristic features;
• which members of a population are vulnerable to deficiency;
• any therapeutic applications of the nutrient;
• what are the gaps in knowledge requiring further study.

12 Carbohydrates in the diet

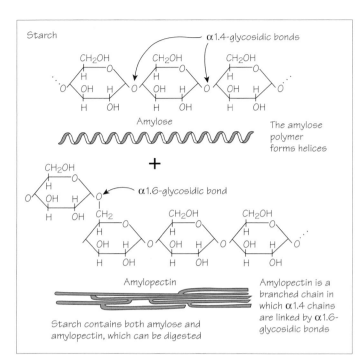

Fig. 12.1 Structures of starches (reproduced with permission from Barasi, M. (2003) *Human Nutrition: A Health Perspective*, Hodder Arnold).

Table 12.1 Classes and fate of carbohydrates in the digestive tract.

Class	Examples	Digestive products
Simple CHOs		
Monosaccharides	Glucose, fructose	Glucose, (some) fructose
Disaccharides	Sucrose	Glucose + fructose
	Lactose	Glucose + galactose
	Maltose	Glucose + glucose
Oligosaccharides	Raffinose	Fermented to short-chain fatty acids (SCFA), hydrogen, methane and carbon dioxide
	Inulin	
Complex CHOs		
Starch	Digestible starch	Glucose
	Resistant starch	Fermented to SCFA, hydrogen, methane and carbon dioxide
Non-starch polysaccharides	Cellulose	Some remain unchanged
	Non-cellulosic polysaccharides, including hemicelluloses, pectins, gums and mucilages	Some fermented to SCFA, hydrogen, methane and carbon dioxide

Aims

(1) To describe the variety of carbohydrates that occur in the human diet, their sources and their fate in the body.

Worldwide, carbohydrates (CHOs) provide 40–80% of the energy consumed by humans, depending on the type of diet; in the UK, CHOs provide in the region of 47% of the energy.

CHOs are classified according to the number of monosaccharide units joined together (polymerised). Three groups are recognised: simple sugars (monosaccharides and disaccharides), oligosaccharides and polysaccharides (Table 12.1).

Monosaccharides

These are simple sugars consisting of 4–6 carbon atoms.

Glucose contains six carbons, and is the commonest sugar in the body. In the diet, it is found in honey, sugar and sugar-based confectionery, cakes, biscuits, fruits and fruit juices and vegetables.

Fructose is found in honey, fruit and some vegetables. Also derived from corn starch, it is now used extensively as a replacement for sucrose in soft drinks, canned fruit, jams and jellies and is present in some dairy products. It is cheaper than sucrose and has better freezing properties. This explains why fructose is now one of the major simple sugars in the Western diet.

After absorption fructose is metabolised in the liver; the products are glucose, glycogen, lactic acid or fat, depending on the metabolic state of the individual.

Galactose is released as a product of the metabolism of lactose from milk. It is essential for neural tissue development in infants and can be transformed into either glucose or glycogen.

Energy plus a healthy bowel

Traditionally it was thought that the major nutritional contribution to health was as an energy source; however, it is now clear that CHOs also play a vital role in the healthy functioning of the bowel.

The use of the terms 'glycaemic' and 'non-glycaemic' carbohydrates encapsulates this difference.

Other monosaccharides

These are occasionally found in foods and include *xylose* and *arabinose* (white wine and beer), *mannose* (fruit) and *fucose* (in human breast milk).

Sorbitol, mannitol and *xylitol* are sugar alcohols, used as sweetening agents in the food industry. They have two valuable properties:

- They are absorbed from the gut and metabolised to glucose more slowly than other simple sugars, delaying the rise in blood glucose, which is of benefit to diabetics.
- They are not fermented by mouth bacteria, and hence do not contribute to dental caries; for this reason they are sometimes added to chewing gum.

Disaccharides

Disaccharides comprise pairs of monosaccharides.

Sucrose is the commonest in the diet, formed by the condensation of glucose and fructose. It is obtained from sugar beet or sugar cane, and by-products of the extraction process include molasses, golden syrup and brown sugar. Sucrose is also found in honey and maple syrup (in solution), fruit and vegetables (associated with the cellular structure).

Lactose consisting of glucose and galactose is present free of cell-wall material in mammalian milk; in the Western diet it originates from cow's milk and its products (e.g. foods containing milk powder or whey such as milk chocolate, muesli, instant potatoes, biscuits and creamed soup). It is widely used by the food industry, and people following a lactose-free diet need to be aware of its prevalence.

Maltose consists of two glucose units and is primarily found in germinating grains such as barley and wheat. The malt produced by this sprouting is used in the production of fermented drinks such as beer. Small amounts of maltose are found in some biscuits, breakfast cereals and malted drinks.

Oligosaccharides

Oligosaccharides, including *stachyose, raffinose* and *inulin*, make a quantitatively small contribution to the diet. They consist of fewer than ten monosaccharide units (generally galactose, maltose or fructose attached to glucose units), and are found in plant foods such as leeks, onions, garlic, Jerusalem artichokes, lentils and beans.

They pass through unchanged to the proximal colon, where they undergo rapid fermentation by bacteria resulting in the production of SCFA and gases, leading to flatulence.

Polysaccharides

Polysaccharides consist of more than ten monosaccharide units arranged in straight, branched or coiled chains. Traditionally divided into digestible (available) forms, such as starches, and non-digestible (unavailable) forms, such as cellulose and lignin, more recently in the UK they have been divided into *starches* and *non-starch polysaccharides* (NSPs), although the term 'dietary fibre' continues to be widely used to encompass the full range of non-digestible CHOs, and includes lignin.

Starch consists of linked glucose units arranged in either straight or branched chains. In *amylose,* there are α1,4-glucosidic bonds linking each of the glucose molecules. *Amylopectin* contains additional α1,6-glucosidic bonds, resulting in a branched structure (Figure 12.1).

Many of the common starchy foods, such as potatoes, cereals and beans, contain amylopectin and amylase in the approximate ratio of 3:1. The relatively high proportion of amylopectin allows starch to form stable gels with good water retention.

Dietary fibre, including non-starch polysaccharides (NSP)

NSPs consist of both cellulose and non-cellulose components, both being polymers of simple sugars.
- Cellulose is the main component of plant cell walls and is made up of many glucose units joined by β1-4 linkages. This makes the molecule very resistant to digestion.
- The non-cellulose polysaccharides consist of the hemicelluloses, pectins, β-glucans, gums and mucilages. They contain sugars such as arabinose, xylose, mannose, fucose, glucose, galactose and rhamnose. These are more readily fermented as a food source for bacteria.

Fructo-oligosaccharides

These consist of fructose residues attached to glucose, and have been developed as potential *prebiotics,* to provide a food source for beneficial bacteria, such as *Bifidobacteria* in the bowel.

Problems with nomenclature

There is confusion in the nomenclature and definition of these CHOs. A number of *analytical methods* have been used that include different components and therefore produce differing values. This causes difficulty both for comparison of research data, and for the consumer, who aspires to eat a 'high-fibre diet'. The methods include:

Southgate method: includes unavailable CHO, lignin and some resistant starch.

Englyst method: assays NSP by a component method and excludes resistant starch.

AOAC: is an enzymatic/gravimetric method that includes both lignin and resistant starch.

13 Carbohydrates in the body

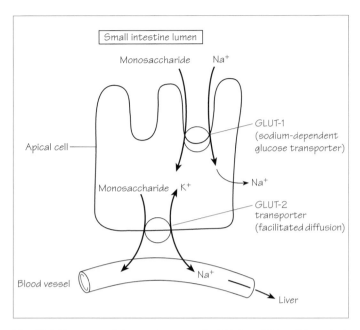

Fig. 13.1 Transport of glucose (monosaccharide) from SI (small intestine) lumen to liver.

Aims

(1) To describe the digestion of carbohydrates.
(2) To introduce the concept of the glycaemic index.

Digestion of carbohydrates

Simple sugars (*monosaccharides*) do not require digestion before absorption, which occurs mainly in the small intestine (SI).

Disaccharides are split by enzymes specific to the particular sugar, as they pass through the mucosal surface of the SI. Deficiencies in these enzymes, most particularly lactase, result in an inability to break down the sugar, and consequent fermentation with associated gas production. Lactase commonly becomes unavailable in individuals who stop consuming milk after infancy, and is widespread in many populations.

Other disaccharidase deficiencies may develop secondary to gastro-intestinal disease, or excess alcohol consumption.

Cooked *starch* is acted on by salivary amylase in the mouth. Low pH levels in the stomach prevent further digestion, but in the duodenum and jejunum, pH levels rise and pancreatic amylase is available, which breaks alternate α1-4 linkages in both raw and cooked starches. Amylose is degraded mostly to maltose and maltotriose with small amounts of glucose released.

Amylopectins are broken down to oligosaccharides, which are subsequently degraded by specific oligosaccharidases bound to the brush border cells, producing glucose as the end product.

Resistant starch (in cell wall material or surrounded by fat in manufactured products) forms a physical barrier slowing access of digestive enzymes to the starch. *Retrograded starches* have been modified

by temperature and/or the formation of a gel, so that on cooling new bonds have formed, resistant to digestion by amylase.

Both resistant and retrograded starches may pass unchanged into the large intestine, where they are fermented by bacteria to SCFA and gases (Table 13.1).

Glucose absorption

Glucose and galactose are transported from the SI across the apical membrane and into the bloodstream by a two-stage mechanism.
• A family of glucose transport proteins is located in cell membranes. Initially glucose moves down its concentration gradient from the SI lumen into apical cells. The Na$^+$-linked transporter GLUT-1 facilitates this diffusion (Figure 13.1).
• Sodium ions are subsequently actively transported out of the apical cell; glucose molecules move from the apical cells into the bloodstream, using the second transport molecule GLUT-2 and facilitated diffusion.

Glycaemic effects of carbohydrates
Glycaemic Index (GI) (Figure 13.2)

The GI provides an indication of how blood glucose levels change after ingesting different carbohydrates. A standard food (usually 50 g of glucose or white bread) is eaten and changes in blood glucose are monitored over a period of time. The effect of a similar amount of the test food is then compared and the GI calculated. Although GI responses can vary between individuals the ranking is similar. It is therefore possible to determine foods which have a low GI and which have a high GI (Table 13.2). Lower GI foods

Table 13.1 Summary of starch digestibility.

Extent of digestion	Food sources
Readily and fully digested	Most cooked starches; sweet potatoes, tapioca
Slowly but completely digested	Flour-based products, e.g. cakes, biscuits, raw cereals
Resistant starch	Green bananas, seeds, cooked and cooled starches; some thickening agents

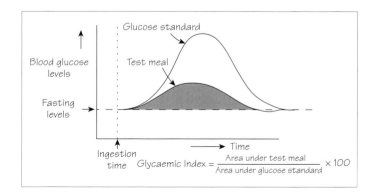

Fig. 13.2 Calculation of Glycaemic Index.

may be preferred in circumstances where a prolonged release of glucose is needed, for example in sporting performance, or to facilitate diabetic blood glucose control. Attention to the GI content of the diet has also recently been recommended for prevention of coronary heart disease, to achieve weight loss and protect against some cancers. However, the evidence for this is still not conclusive.

It should be remembered that GI values for single foods may not be replicated for whole meals, and depend on the dietary mix.

Non-glycaemic effects of carbohydrates

Diets rich in NSP encourage chewing, which both slows the process of eating and increases saliva flow, contributing to satiation and promoting dental health.

As NSP travels through the SI, divalent cations such as calcium, zinc and iron are bound to the surface of the NSP, which may reduce their availability for absorption.

In the large intestine *soluble fibre* is acted upon by the bacterial flora; this process of fermentation releases a number of SCFA: propionic and acetic acids are metabolised in the liver but butyric acid is used locally by gut colonocytes as an essential source of energy. The multiplication of the bacterial flora increases bulk and water content of the stools.

Insoluble fibre reaches the colon largely unchanged and is not fermented by bacteria. The water-holding characteristics of insoluble fibre mean that together with the large bacterial mass, the total intra-colonic mass is greater and leads to increased peristaltic action, which increases the speed of movement of the colon contents. This action reduces overall transit time through the gastrointestinal tract, and contributes to the overall laxation effect.

The range of CHOs consumed provides the body not only with glucose to maintain blood levels of this essential nutrient for brain and nervous system function, but also a food source for colonic bacteria, which enables a population of beneficial microorganisms to be maintained in the colon, contributing to colon health.

Table 13.2 Glycaemic Index of some common foods.

Foods with high GI (>85)	Foods with moderate GI (60–85)	Foods with low GI (<60)
Bread (white or wholemeal)	Pasta and noodles	Apples, grapefruit, peaches, plums
Rice	Porridge	Beans
Breakfast cereals, e.g. muesli, Weetabix	Grapes, oranges	Milk, yogurt, ice cream
Raisins, bananas	Crisps	Fructose
Potatoes, sweetcorn	Biscuits	Tomato soup
Glucose, sucrose, honey		
Soft drinks		

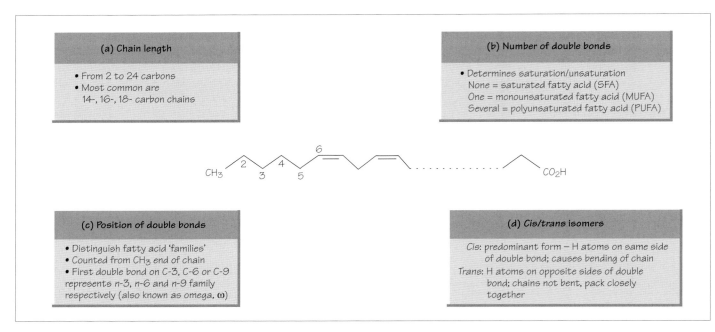

(a) Chain length

- From 2 to 24 carbons
- Most common are 14-, 16-, 18- carbon chains

(b) Number of double bonds

- Determines saturation/unsaturation
  None = saturated fatty acid (SFA)
  One = monounsaturated fatty acid (MUFA)
  Several = polyunsaturated fatty acid (PUFA)

(c) Position of double bonds

- Distinguish fatty acid 'families'
- Counted from CH_3 end of chain
- First double bond on C-3, C-6 or C-9 represents n-3, n-6 and n-9 family respectively (also known as omega, ω)

(d) Cis/trans isomers

Cis: predominant form – H atoms on same side of double bond; causes bending of chain
Trans: H atoms on opposite sides of double bond; chains not bent, pack closely together

Fig. 14.1 Causes of variation between fatty acids.

Aims

(1) To consider the fats that are common in the diet.
(2) To describe specific nutritional characteristics of fatty acids.

Major roles of fats

Fats (or lipids) are essential in the diet to provide:

- a concentrated source of energy (providing 37 kJ/g, or 9 kcal/g);
- an insulating layer under the skin;
- structural components in the body;
- functional constituents of many metabolic processes;
- a vehicle for intake and absorption of fat-soluble vitamins;
- an important contributor to flavour and palatability of foods.
  The most important lipids in nutrition are:

- *Triacylglycerols* (TAGs, also known as triglycerides): these contain three fatty acids attached to a molecule of glycerol; comprise up to 95% of dietary lipids.
- *Phospholipids*: contain a glycerol backbone, with two fatty acids (nonpolar) and a 'polar head group' with a phosphoric acid residue and either sugars or amino acids. The commonest example is phosphatidylcholine (lecithin). Phospholipids have an amphipathic nature and can act at the interface between aqueous and lipid environments. This also allows them to function as emulsifying agents.

- *Sterols*: contain carbon, hydrogen and oxygen arranged as ring structures, with associated side chains. Cholesterol is the main sterol in animal tissues, often associated with a fatty acid, forming cholesteryl esters. Plants contain phytosterols.

Fat-soluble vitamins are associated with these lipids.

Fatty acids are the main components of dietary lipids. Their generic structure has a carbon backbone, with a carboxyl (–COOH) group at one end and a methyl group (–CH3) at the other end.

The fatty acids differ from one another in a number of ways (Figure 14.1). These variations result in a diversity of physical properties of the fatty acids and therefore the resulting lipids, affecting their metabolic role and consequences for health.

Saturated fatty acids (SFAs)

These contain the maximum number of hydrogen atoms on each carbon, and tend to be solid at room temperature.

Short notation for fatty acids

The differences in structure can be summarised in a short notation for the fatty acid, as illustrated by two examples:

C18:2, *n*-6 is linoleic acid, with 18 carbons, two double bonds, the first of which starts on the sixth carbon from the methyl end of the acid.

C18:3, *n*-3 is α-linolenic acid, with 18 carbons, three double bonds, the first of which starts on the third carbon from the methyl end of the acid.

Fats and disease

The intake of dietary fats and their composition have been the subjects of extensive research, because of the involvement of fats in certain diseases, such as cardiovascular disease and cancers, as well as having a potential role in the development of obesity.

- Milk fat, containing SFAs synthesised by rumen bacteria, is the main dietary source of short- and medium-chain SFAs, with four to ten carbons. Products such as butter are rich in these fatty acids.
- The majority of SFAs in the diet contain 14, 16 and 18 carbons, and come from palm (C16) and coconut oil (C14), animal and hydrogenated fats.
- Longer chain SFAs, up to 24 carbons, are synthesised within brain tissue membranes.

Monounsaturated fatty acids (MUFAs)

- These contain one double bond, with the main example being oleic acid (18:1, *n*-9), derived from olive and rapeseed oils.
- MUFAs from oily fish may also be present in small amounts.
- In India, mustard seed oil provides erucic acid (22:1, *n*-9).

Polyunsaturated fatty acids (PUFAs)

PUFAs have the lowest melting point of all the types of fatty acids, because of the presence of double bonds. They are liquid at room temperature; when used in the manufacture of spreading fats, emulsification is used to produce a more solid spread.

- The major PUFAs contain 18–22 carbons, up to six double bonds and belong to the *n*-3 and *n*-6 families.
- PUFAs and their derivatives regulate fluidity and other properties of membranes, with a particular role in the brain, nervous system and retina for the *n*-3 PUFAs.
- They are also used in the formation of *eicosanoids* (metabolic regulators), including prostaglandins, prostacyclins, thromboxanes and leukotrienes. Eicosanoids from the *n*-3 and *n*-6 families differ

in their potency and functions, and an altered balance between these can affect functions such as haemostasis and inflammation.

The body is unable to synthesise the parent compounds of the *n*-3 and *n*-6 PUFAs, and these are termed the *essential fatty acids*, which must be supplied in the diet. In the body, the parent acid can be converted into longer chain forms. This occurs by a series of desaturation (adding a double bond by removing hydrogen) and elongation (adding two carbon atoms) reactions (Figure 14.2).

Trans fatty acids (TFAs)

Unsaturated fatty acids can contain one or more double bonds arranged in the *trans* position. Meat and milk from ruminant animals, and hydrogenated fats are both potential sources of TFAs. These have characteristics similar to SFAs, as a result of closer alignment of molecules.

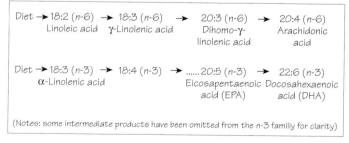

Fig. 14.2 Interconversions between fatty acids within families.

15 Introduction to fats: related compounds and fat digestion

Aims

(1) To consider the nutritional role of phospholipids and sterols.
(2) To summarise how the body digests and absorbs dietary fat.

Phospholipids and sterols are present in small amounts in the diet, but play a vital role in the structure and function of the body.

Cholesterol

This is the principal sterol found in the body.

• It is synthesised from acetyl coenzyme A, in all tissues but mainly in the liver.

• It plays a key role in membrane structure and transport across the membrane, and in the synthesis of hormones and bile acids.

• Animal foods are the source of dietary cholesterol, with egg yolk being the richest source. Absorption of cholesterol is variable, but generally less than 50%. Plasma levels, principally carried in the LDL fraction, are major determinants of the risk of atherosclerosis.

Phospholipids

These are found widely in the diet, albeit in small amounts, as they form essential components of cell membranes.

• Liver and eggs are important sources from animal foods; soya bean and wheatgerm are rich plant sources (Table 15.1).

Lower cholesterol?

Healthy eating advice has principally been focused on dietary modification to reduce plasma LDL levels. However, it must be noted that there is genetic variability in LDL levels and their response to dietary cholesterol intakes, such that reductions in dietary cholesterol are no longer considered a major part of dietary advice for most people.

Phytosterols are derived from plants; β-sitosterol is obtained from nuts, cereals and fats and oils. Plant stanol (saturated) and sterol (unsaturated) esters have been marketed in recent years to help in cholesterol lowering, as they compete with cholesterol for absorption and promote the increased loss of cholesterol in the faeces. An intake of 2 g/day of these compounds appears to have the optimal effect.

Table 15.1 Summary of the occurrence of main types of fat in the diet.

Type of fat	Main dietary sources
Short-chain SFA (C4–C10)	Milk, milk products and butter
SFAs with 14–18 carbons	Meat, animal foods and fats Coconut and palm oils
MUFAs, especially C18:1	Olive and rapeseed oils
PUFAs, *n*-6	Specific fatty acids from this family occur as follows: Linoleic acid: seed oils (sunflower, soya bean and corn), meat, eggs and nuts γ-Linolenic acid: borage, blackcurrant and evening primrose oil Arachidonic acid: small amounts in meat and egg yolks
PUFAs, *n*-3	Specific fatty acids from this family occur as follows: α-Linolenic acid: dark-green vegetables, meat from grass-fed ruminants, seed oils (flaxseed, soya bean and rapeseed) Eicosapentaenoic acid (EPA) and docosahexaenoic acid (DHA): oily fish and fish oils
Cholesterol	Foods of animal origin: eggs, organ meats, shellfish
Phospholipids	Small amounts in soya bean, wheatgerm oils; animal foods, eggs
TFAs	Products from ruminant animals; hydrogenated fats in manufactured goods

• Within the body, phospholipids are found in all cell membranes, where they contribute to structural integrity, but are also an important source of essential fatty acids for the local production of eicosanoids.

Fat digestion and absorption

In order that dietary fat is effectively processed in the digestive tract, a number of difficulties associated with digestion of fat need to be overcome (Table 15.2).

Fat intake and diet

Fat is perceived by many people as the component of the diet to be reduced as much as possible. However, this is not conducive to health, as a certain amount of fat, usually around 30% of the total energy, is required to fulfil the important roles that fat has in the body. Diets that are low in fat can be very bulky, as the energy density is reduced, and more food has to be consumed to achieve an adequate energy intake. When consumers wish to reduced their energy consumption, reducing their fat intake can be helpful, but under these circumstances it is important to ensure that essential fatty acids and fat-soluble vitamins are still being supplied to meet nutritional requirements.

Table 15.2 Obstacles to fat digestion and their physiological solutions.

Problem	Solution	Consequences
Dietary fat is not miscible with aqueous digestive juices	Large fat particles broken down in stomach by churning action	Coarse emulsion reaches duodenum Hormones (e.g. cholecystokinin) released to slow down stomach emptying and promote release of bile
Digestive enzymes cannot process large lipids	Bile released from liver, via gall bladder, reduces the coarse emulsion to small micelles, which can be acted on by pancreatic lipase	Lipase splits fatty acids from TAGs to yield glycerol, fatty acids and some monoacylglycerols
Some digestion products are too large to enter directly into circulation. Short- and medium-chain fatty acids can be absorbed directly	Packaged into chylomicrons, where hydrophilic constituents form the outer coat and hydrophobic products are in the interior. Bile acids are reabsorbed from the ileum and recirculated	Chylomicrons pass into the lymphatic system draining the digestive tract for carriage to the peripheral circulation, which they enter at the thoracic duct

16 Fats: utilisation in the body

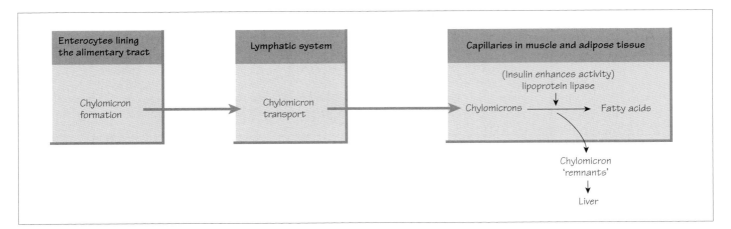

Fig. 16.1 Transport of fats to tissues.

Aims

(1) To consider how fats are transported in the body.
(2) To study fat storage and utilisation.

Transport of fats in the body: lipoproteins

Because fats are hydrophobic, they cannot circulate freely in the blood, but are packaged into several aggregate particles, known as lipoproteins. The composition of lipoproteins is dynamic (i.e. not constant) as constituents are taken up and released (Table 16.1).

The main function of lipoproteins is to transport Triacylglycerol (TAG) and cholesterol originating from the diet or endogenous synthesis. These particles also carry other fat-soluble materials. Proteins, known as apolipoproteins, serve as 'identifiers' for the particles, and determine their uptake by receptor sites.

Chylomicrons

These are the largest and lightest of the lipoproteins, and transport exogenous TAG taken in from the diet. They peak in the circulation 2–4 hours after a fat-containing meal, but may continue to enter for up to 14 hours after a particularly high-fat meal. They release fatty acids as they travel through the body, and their 'remnants' are taken up by the liver.

Table 16.1 Typical composition of lipoprotein particles (as percentage).

Particle	Triacylglycerol (TAG)	Cholesterol	Phospholipid	Protein
Chylomicron	90	5	3	2
Very low-density lipoprotein (VLDL)	60	12	18	10
Low-density lipoprotein (LDL)	10	50	15	25
High-density lipoprotein (HDL)	5	20	25	50

The current needs of the body, for immediate energy (in muscle) or storage (in adipose tissues), determine at which sites lipoprotein lipase (LPL) is most active and fatty acids are released (Figure 16.1).

Very low-density lipoproteins (VLDLs)

These are made in the liver by the resynthesis of TAG from fatty acids delivered to the liver. Peak release of VLDLs from the liver occurs 2–3 hours after a meal, but if chylomicrons are still present, these are preferentially metabolised.

As VLDL lose TAG, their cholesterol concentration rises, and they become low-density lipoproteins (LDLs).

Low-density lipoproteins (LDLs)

The principal function of LDLs is to transport cholesterol to tissues where it is needed in cell membranes and for synthesis of metabolites, such as steroid hormones. LDL receptors recognise apoB100 on LDLs; receptor activity is regulated by intracellular free cholesterol levels. Thus, LDL uptake can be varied to meet cellular needs for cholesterol (Figure 16.2).

High-density lipoproteins (HDLs)

HDLs are synthesised in the intestines and the liver. They collect free cholesterol from the peripheral tissues. This is esterified by LCAT to cholesterol esters (CE), to maintain a concentration gradient into the HDL.

• The CE may be taken directly to the liver and excreted in bile, or exchanged for TAG from VLDLs and chylomicrons. If this happens to excess, TAG-rich HDLs (small dense HDLs) become a substrate for hepatic lipase, when they are rapidly catabolised; this may lead to lower circulating levels of HDLs.

• This then reduces the normal reverse cholesterol transport process, and cholesterol levels in the tissues may increase.

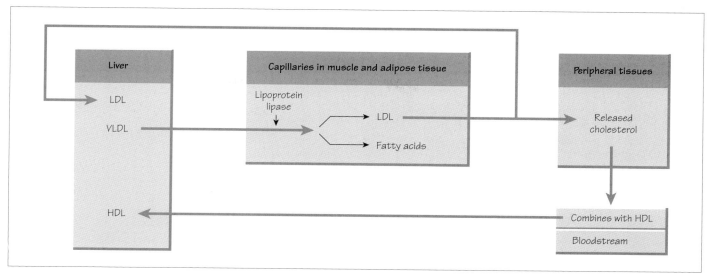

Fig. 16.2 Summary of lipid transport.

Because LDLs and HDLs are intimately involved with cholesterol transport they are believed to be critical in the development of atherosclerosis and heart disease.

Adipose tissue

Fat is stored as an energy reserve in adipocytes, found in adipose tissue. These cells make up only about half of the total cell numbers within the tissue: fibroblasts, macrophages and vascular tissue make up the remainder. Adipose tissue itself contains approximately 79% fat, 18% water and 3% protein.

• *White adipose tissue* is the predominant form; the cells store fat as a single droplet, which fills almost the entire cell. The type of fat reflects the type of dietary fat consumed: on a low-fat diet, the fat is mainly that synthesised in the body, containing mainly palmitic, stearic and oleic acids.

• There are also small amounts of *brown adipose tissue* (BAT), mostly found in young children, but possibly also in adults. BAT has many more mitochondria, blood capillaries and nerve fibres than white adipose tissue. In young children and animals, BAT is a means of generating heat. It may play some role in energy wasting mechanisms in adults and so help in energy balance.

Amounts of fat stored

The healthy adult male contains about 17% of his weight as fat, the female approximately 27%. The majority of this fat is found subcutaneously. Deposits within the chest cavity and abdomen increase with fatness, and are associated with increased health risks.

Mobilisation of stored fat

There are differences between abdominal fat and that stored in the thighs and buttocks.

• Intra-abdominal fat is more sensitive to lipolytic stimuli, and the fat released in this region is carried directly to the liver in the portal vein, triggering metabolic responses.

• Subcutaneous fat is more resistant to lipolysis and is more likely to be protected from daily fluctuations.

• Fat adjacent to lymph nodes is thought to support the immune system, and may expand in chronic inflammatory states, at the expense of fat in other regions.

Metabolism of stored fat

Fat storage and release is under hormonal control, principally insulin and noradrenaline. There is a continuous flux of fats into and out of the adipocytes.

Fat storage occurs principally in the postprandial phase under the influence of insulin, when there are increased numbers of chylomicrons and VLDLs in the circulation.

In theory fat can be synthesised from carbohydrates for storage, but this rarely happens, except in circumstances of very high carbohydrate intake. Thus most fat stored is derived from dietary and endogenous fats.

Fat utilisation occurs under the influence of noradrenaline, which causes the release of fatty acids and their oxidation to yield ATP. Some fat oxidation occurs most of the time in the human body to fuel metabolic and physical activity.

Adipose tissue has other functions including:

• Sectretion of leptin.

• Release of proteins involved in blood pressure regulation.

• Production of cytokines and other immune active factors.

Loss of control

As body fat levels increase, there is a reduced ability of adipose tissue to respond to regulatory signals, with an increase in circulating lipid levels and the risk of fat depositing in liver and skeletal muscle.

Insulin resistance is a feature, and the disposal of glucose is also affected. Type 2 diabetes may result and be accompanied by a range of complications, including hypertension, damage to peripheral blood vessels, hyperlipidaemia and risk of cardiovascular disease.

17 Proteins: chemistry and digestion

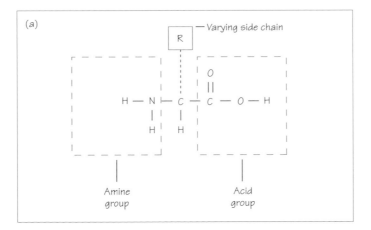

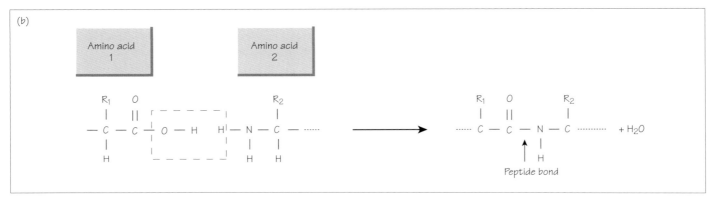

Fig. 17.1 (a) Generic structure of amino acid. (b) Condensation of two amino acids to form dipeptide.

Aims

(1) To describe the basic structure of proteins.
(2) To consider how proteins are digested.

Proteins form the basic building blocks of all living cells (i.e. found in cell membranes and organelles), as well as the enzymes and chemical messengers that integrate body functions.

In contrast to carbohydrates and fats, which contain only carbon, hydrogen and oxygen, proteins also contain nitrogen and are the most abundant nitrogen-containing molecules in the body.

Structure of proteins

A protein molecule is made up of a chain of *individual amino acids*, linked by peptide bonds. The chain becomes folded in various ways and links are made between amino acids that come to lie adjacent to each other, commonly by hydrogen bonds between oxygen and nitrogen atoms, or by interactions between side chains.

Folding and cross-linking contributes:
- strength and elasticity to particular structural proteins;
- reactive sites for receptors or enzymic activity.

Amino acids

The sequence in which amino acids are present determines the iden-

tity and function of a protein. There are 20 amino acids, in combinations ranging from 50 to over 1000 in any one protein, contributing to enormous diversity.

Amino acids have a common basic structure, as shown in Figure 17.1, with varying side chains. Side chains may be hydrophilic or hydrophobic, as well as aliphatic, aromatic, acidic or basic, resulting in amino acids with these properties, as shown in Table 17.1.

Digestion and absorption of proteins

In their native form, most proteins are very resistant to digestion, with only the superficial bonds susceptible to proteolytic activity. However, once a protein has been denatured, by exposure to either heat or acid, the forces holding the structure together become weakened, and digestion can occur. Cooking and the acidity of stomach contents both contribute to increasing the digestibility of proteins.

Enzymes are secreted as inactive *proenzymes* (*zymogens*), and activated only after secretion into the stomach or duodenum; this protects the organs from autodigestion by proteolytic enzymes.

The polypeptide chains are broken at specific sites, exposing more terminal sites for further cleavage. In this way, progressively shorter peptide chains are produced.

Table 17.1 Classification of amino acids.

Aromatic	Aliphatic	Acidic	Basic
Phenylalanine	Glycine	Aspartic acid	Lysine
Tyrosine	Alanine	Asparagine	Arginine
Tryptophan	Valine[a]	Glutamic acid	Histidine
	Leucine[a]	Glutamine	
	Isoleucine[a]		
	Serine		
	Threonine		
	Cysteine[b]		
	Cystine[b]		
	Methionine[b]		
	Proline		

[a]Branched-chain amino acids.

[b]Sulphur-containing amino acids.

Overall, the process liberates free amino acids as well as other small peptides, which are themselves further split by aminopeptidases located within the intestinal mucosa during the process of absorption. Protein digestion is summarised in Table 17.2.

Dietary protein is normally almost completely digested. However, the presence of indigestible cell walls and trypsin inhibitors (in raw beans) will interfere with the process. In general, legumes are considered the least effectively digested protein source.

Absorption occurs both by passive diffusion and by sodium-dependent active transport mechanisms. Some intact protein may be absorbed, which can give rise to allergic reactions (see Chapter 47), although it is important in very young infants, where it confers some immunity (see Chapter 39). Absorbed amino acids enter the circulation via the portal vein.

In addition to the dietary amino acids presented for absorption, the intestinal mucosa also absorbs considerable amounts of endogenous amino acids (approximately 80 g/day), derived from secretions into the small intestine, and cells sloughed off the mucosal surface.

Table 17.2 Summary of protein digestion.

Organ/site	Secretion(s)	Action and products
Mouth/teeth/chewing action	Saliva	Lubricates food, allows breakdown to smaller pieces
Stomach	Hydrochloric acid (HCl) Pepsinogen	HCl: –denatures proteins –activates pepsinogen to pepsin at pH <4 Pepsin: –breaks polypeptide chains to smaller units → shorter polypeptides
Pancreas	Bicarbonate Pancreatic enzymes: –trypsinogen[a] –chymotrypsinogen –carboxypeptidases –endopeptidases[a]	Bicarbonate: –increases pH (to approx. 7.5) to allow enzymes to work Trypsin (formed from trypsinogen): –cleaves polypeptides with basic terminal amino acid –activates other proteolytic enzymes Chymotrypsin: –cleaves polypeptides with a neutral terminal amino acid Carboxypeptidases: –remove successive amino acids from carboxy terminal of peptide chain Endopeptidases: –attack bonds within the peptide chain
Small intestine	Enterokinase (also called enteropeptidase) Aminopeptidases	Enterokinase: –activates trypsin and endopeptidases Aminopeptidases: –complete breakdown of small peptide chains (tri- and dipeptides) as they pass through the intestinal mucosa

[a]Activated by enterokinase from small intestine.

18 Proteins: functions in the body

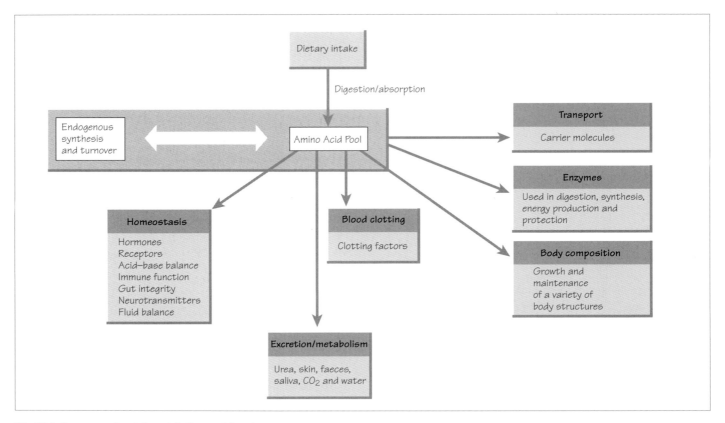

Fig. 18.1 Summary of protein metabolism and function.

Aims

(1) To identify the main functions of proteins in the body.
(2) To recognise the role of essential amino acids in protein function and metabolism.

The amino acids from the digestive tract enter the 'amino acid pool' and are used to synthesise proteins required for various functions in the body. The metabolism and functions of proteins are summarised in Figure 18.1.

Metabolism of amino acids
Protein synthesis and breakdown

There is a continuous turnover of protein in the body, which in healthy adults exhibits a balance between synthesis and breakdown, and amounts to 3–6 g/kg body weight per day.

During growth there is an excess of synthesis over breakdown, and in wasting conditions (e.g. starvation, cancer and after surgery or trauma), breakdown exceeds synthesis.

Protein synthesis is regulated principally by insulin, and catabolism by glucocorticoids. At the cellular level, the transcription of DNA into messenger RNA (mRNA) forms the template for protein synthesis on the ribosome.

Essential and nonessential amino acids (see Table 18.1)

• The body is unable to make nine of the amino acids used in protein

Table 18.1 Essential and nonessential amino acids.

Indispensable amino acids (essential)	Conditionally indispensable (or essential) amino acids	Dispensable (or nonessential) amino acids
Histidine	Arginine	Alanine
Isoleucine	Cysteine	Aspartate
Leucine	Glutamine	Asparagine
Lysine	Glycine	Glutamate
Methionine	Proline	Serine
Phenylalanine	Tyrosine	
Threonine		
Tryptophan		
Valine		

synthesis, and these must be supplied by the diet, or derived from breakdown of other proteins. These are known as the 'essential' or 'indispensable' amino acids. Lack of any one of these will limit the synthesis of protein, even if all the other required amino acids are present in adequate amounts.

• In addition, there are a number of other amino acids that can be synthesised in the body under normal conditions, given the necessary supply of precursor molecules. In the absence of these precursors, the amino acids become 'conditionally indispensable'. This is also the case in prematurity and in disease or physiological stress, where the

capacity for synthesis is outstripped by the need for the amino acid.
• The remaining amino acids can be made from metabolic intermediates that are not limiting, and so are not required to be supplied as such by the diet.

Utilisation of amino acids

Protein synthesis is an energy-demanding process; it has been calculated that the energy requirement is 4.2 kJ (1 kcal)/g of protein synthesised. Protein synthesis occurs more rapidly after a meal than in the fasting state, due to the greater supply of amino acids. On average the energy used in protein synthesis accounts for 12% of the basal metabolic rate.

Some amino acids are used for the synthesis of other molecules (Table 18.2). These molecules regulate vital functions in the body and represent a substantial proportion of the daily turnover of specific amino acids.

Oxidation of amino acids

There is no functional store of amino acids, so those that are not used directly, or indirectly (by conversion to another amino acid where possible) are oxidised. This process can be considered in two parts.
(1) Removal of the amino group initially yields ammonia, which is converted to urea in the liver; some of this is excreted via the kidneys, but the remainder is reabsorbed into the colon from the bloodstream, and recycled by the bacteria to carbon dioxide and ammonia, which can be used for the synthesis of nitrogenous compounds. This cycle is termed *urea salvage*.
(2) The carbon skeleton of the amino acid is ultimately converted to carbon dioxide and water, with the release of ATP. This occurs particularly in the liver, which obtains a major part of its fuel needs from this oxidation.

Glutamine breakdown is a major source of fuel for the gut and white blood cells.

The final pathway by which the carbon skeletons of amino acids are utilised depends on their structure. The majority are metabolised to

Table 18.2 Use of amino acid for synthesis of derived products.

Amino acid	Product	Function
Arginine	Nitric oxide	Leucocyte function, vascular tone, neurotransmitter
	Creatine	Energy production
Glycine	Haem	Oxygen transport
	Creatine	Energy production
Tyrosine	Hormones: thyroid, melanin	Homeostasis
	Neurotransmitters (adrenaline, noradrenaline, dopamine)	Neuronal integration
Tryptophan	Nicotinic acid	Vitamin function
	Serotonin (5-hydroxytryptamine)	Transmitter function
Histidine	Histamine	Transmitter; inflammatory response
Lysine	Carnitine	Lipid metabolism
Cysteine, glutamate and glycine	Glutathione	Antioxidant role
Methionine	Creatine	Energy production
Glutamine	Nucleotides	Cell division
	Glutathione	Antioxidant role

glucose and are termed *glucogenic*. *Ketogenic* amino acids (including leucine and lysine) give rise to acetoacetic acid and ultimately yield acetyl CoA. A few of the amino acids may be both glucogenic and ketogenic, including tryptophan, methionine, cysteine, phenylalanine, tyrosine and isoleucine.

Conclusion

Proteins are essential for life, but it is the amino acids that they contain that are the key to their functions. These are released from food and utilised efficiently in the body, to fulfil a broad range of functions. Protein needs are considered in Chapter 19.

19 Proteins: needs and sources

Aims

(1) To quantify the body's need for protein.
(2) To identify sources of protein and how these fulfil protein needs.

The need for protein

Protein is required for maintenance of the body's structure and functions at all times. Extra protein may be required during growth, in pregnancy and repair after injury.

Establishing how much protein is required is problematic, for three reasons:

- Protein deficiency, which would be used as a basis for quantifying the requirement, is a nonspecific condition, affecting many processes, is difficult to define and therefore cannot be used as a baseline.
- The body is able to adapt to varying levels of protein intake, and protein metabolism is affected by levels of energy intake.
- The methods available are imprecise, and rely on balance studies, which rarely include all constituents of protein flux.

Nitrogen balance

Protein metabolism in the body has traditionally been extrapolated from nitrogen intake and loss to provide a measure of 'nitrogen balance'.

Nitrogen balance is the difference between the intake and losses of nitrogen.

- A *positive nitrogen balance* implies that protein is being utilised and retained in the body, in growth or major tissue repair. Nitrogen balance does not become positive simply as a result of an increased dietary intake of protein; the extra protein may be used for energy, and the excess nitrogen excreted as urea.
- A *negative nitrogen balance*, where losses exceed intake, is indicative of protein breakdown and may be the result of starvation, injury or a catabolic state. It may also occur with low energy intakes when protein is used for energy rather than maintenance and repair.

Using nitrogen measurement to assess balance assumes that all protein has 16% nitrogen content, so that a value obtained for nitrogen flux can be converted to a protein flux using the factor of 6.25 (100/16). It excludes non-protein nitrogenous sources, which may be significant.

There are *inherent difficulties* in measuring nitrogen loss. Nitrogen is lost in:

- urine (as urea, uric acid, creatinine, ammonium compounds);
- faeces (unabsorbed nitrogen, bacterial protein);
- skin, hair, nails, saliva and sweat, breath and colonic gases (all of these are difficult to quantify).

On the basis of such measurement, it has been calculated that when the diet is totally devoid of protein, the daily nitrogen losses amount to 55 mg/kg body weight, which is equivalent to a protein loss of 0.34 g/kg body weight.

Methods of assessing protein quality

Digestibility (expressed as N)

This represents the proportion of nitrogen that is *absorbed from ingested foods,* and is expressed as the amount of N absorbed as a proportion of the N intake. The amount absorbed is obtained by subtracting the amount excreted in the faeces from the amount eaten.

(Note: the amount excreted also includes nitrogen from intestinal secretions, intestinal cells and bacteria, and for accuracy these should be taken into account. Measurements using radioactively labelled nitrogen suggest that up to 50% of faecal N may be of endogenous origin.)

- The digestibility of proteins from animal sources is much greater than that from plant sources. Digestibility for egg is given as 97%.
- Poor digestibility, of between 60 and 80%, is found in legumes and cereals with tough cell walls, particularly when uncooked, and is a factor in diets that are low in protein.

Net protein utilisation (NPU)

This measures the *nitrogen retention* in the body in relation to the intake, and thus includes a measure of nitrogen losses in the urine as well as those in the faeces. It can be measured in human volunteers, fed specific sources of protein over test periods. NPU can then be expressed as:

$$NPU = \frac{nitrogen\ retained \times 100}{nitrogen\ intake}$$

(where nitrogen retained is: N intake – urine N – faecal N (adjusted for endogenous loss)).

Individual proteins give a range of NPU values when tested separately:

Maize	36
Wheat	49
Rice	63
Soya	67
Cow's milk	81
Egg	87

However, in practice, unless these sources represent the only protein in the diet, combinations of protein sources can increase the amount of N retained (see below).

Biological value (BV)

This measures the $\dfrac{N\ retained \times 100}{N\ absorbed}$

This calculation takes into account the digestibility and is a better measure of the effectiveness of the protein to meet the body's needs.

BV is 100 for egg protein, and 75 for beef and fish; values above 70 are considered to reflect protein quality sufficient to maintain growth.

This is termed the *obligatory loss*. When the efficiency of utilisation is taken into account, a daily figure of 0.66 g/kg body weight as a maintenance requirement is obtained.

Assessing protein quality

Proteins consumed in the diet must be converted into the proteins typically found in the human body, to fulfil physiological needs.

Protein quality can be defined as the efficiency with which a protein can be utilised by the body. Accordingly, various ways exist of evaluating the quality of proteins in terms of meeting these needs. None of these give a completely satisfactory assessment of protein quality, and new methods continue to be developed.

Amino acid score

The supply of amino acids in correct proportions for the body's needs is the fundamental determinant of protein quality. For a protein to be useful it must provide the *essential amino acids* in the appropriate amounts (nonessential amino acids can be synthesised from other amino acids as required).

Synthesis of any new proteins can only occur up to the limit of the essential amino acid present in the least amount relative to its need. This is termed the *limiting amino acid*. Thus for all of the essential amino acids in a protein, an 'amino acid score' can be calculated, with the lowest score indicating the limiting amino acid.

A *protein-digestibility-corrected amino acid score* (PDCAAS), developed by the FAO, gives the most accurate calculated values.

In practice, lysine is the common limiting amino acid in cereals, sulphur amino acids (methionine and cystine) in legumes, and occasionally tryptophan or threonine. However, when people consume mixed diets, as is normally the case, the combinations of foods provide sufficient amino acids at the same time to compensate for shortages in particular food groups (Table 19.1).

Recommended intakes for protein

The UK's Department of Health (DoH) 1991 recommendations (see Appendix 3) use the safe level of intake of 0.75 g/kg body weight, to establish the Reference Nutrient Intake (RNI) for protein; this equals 56 g/day for an adult male and 45 g/day for a female.

These values represent approximately 8–9% of the total energy intake. Both of these values are lower than the amounts of protein

Table 19.1 Use of food combinations to compensate for limiting amino acid.

Plant food	Limiting amino acid	Useful complementary food	Example of meal
Grains or cereals	Lysine, threonine	Legumes, pulses	Beans on toast Pasta and beans
Nuts and seeds	Lysine	Legumes, pulses	Hummus (chickpeas with sesame seeds)
Soya beans and other legumes/pulses	Methionine	Grains, nuts and seeds	Lentil curry and rice Couscous and beans
Maize	Tryptophan, lysine	Legumes	Tortillas and beans
Vegetables	Methionine	Grains, nuts and seeds	Vegetable and nut stew

actually consumed in the UK, which reaches up to 15% of the energy consumed, with a mean intake of approximately 67 g.

Protein requirements are greater in:
• patients recovering from major disease;
• athletes in training, who may require a larger amount of protein expressed per kilogram body weight (see Chapter 45).

Excessively high protein intakes may contribute to kidney disease or bone demineralisation, but evidence for this is equivocal. However, intakes at 1.5 g/kg body weight are considered to be the safe upper limit.

Dietary protein sources

Worldwide, the availability of plant proteins is relatively consistent, at about 50 g/person/day. However, the availability of animal protein sources varies widely, from <5 to 50 g/head/day, highest in most Western countries.

The supply of protein in relation to energy is generally 10–12%, with some exceptions where protein-poor staples, such as cassava and plantain, are eaten.

Deficiency of protein

Inadequate protein intakes rarely occur alone, and are generally found within a wider picture of undernutrition.

Insufficient intakes of energy cause protein to be used for energy, and make it unavailable for tissue maintenance or growth.

In *children,* there is stunted growth, muscle wasting, poor wound healing and increased risk of infection. Plasma albumin levels will be low, resulting in oedema. The classical description of this syndrome is *kwashiorkor,* although it is considered that other deficiencies, of fatty acids and minerals, contribute to the overall picture.

In *hospital malnutrition syndrome,* patients may have increased needs due to injury, trauma and the need for tissue repair, but are unable to consume sufficient nutrients. In a process driven by cytokines, protein is broken down in muscle to provide amino acids for the immune system and the synthesis of acute-phase proteins in the liver. The synthesis of normal transport proteins in the liver may be reduced. There is an overall negative nitrogen balance; the extent varies depending on the magnitude of the trauma, but may represent protein losses of 5–70 g/day.

There are a number of implications of hospital malnutrition syndrome that affect the outcome for the patient. These include:
• Increased risk of complications and poor wound healing.
• Poor immune status and risk of infection.
• Reduced muscle strength, inability to swallow and cough.
• Apathy, depression and reduced quality of life.
Attention to nutritional support can minimise these risks.

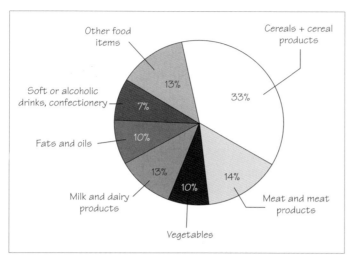

Fig. 20.1 Contribution of major food groups to energy intakes in the UK.

Aims

(1) To describe how energy intake from food is quantified.
(2) To identify the main food groups contributing to energy intake.

Energy is needed for all the functions performed by the body. These include:
• metabolic activity at cellular, tissue and organ level, which is largely outside our conscious awareness and continues throughout life;

Units used for measuring energy in nutrition

Traditionally, the unit of measurement of energy in nutrition has been the kilocalorie (kcal or Calorie), reflecting the observed generation of heat by metabolic reactions.

More recently, the kilojoule (kJ), the unit for measurement of energy, has been preferred by nutritionists. Both units are used, and in general members of the public recognise kilocalories rather than kilojoules.

It is therefore essential to know the conversion factor between the two units:

1 kilocalorie = 4.18 kilojoules.

Larger amounts of energy may be expressed in terms of megajoules (MJ), where 1 MJ = 1000 kJ.

Methods for measuring food energy

The potential energy contained in food can be measured using a bomb calorimeter, which combusts the food in the presence of oxygen to release its energy. This value is the *gross energy*. However, the breakdown of food in the body, during digestion, absorption and metabolism, is not so efficient, and the energy available at the biochemical level is therefore less than that obtained by combustion. This is known as the *metabolisable energy*, which represents the energy actually supplied to the tissues by each food.

The amount of metabolisable energy available from each macronutrient is known from meticulous studies, and these values (known as proximate principles or *energy conversion factors*) are used in the calculation of the energy content of foods, as found in food composition tables (Table 20.1).

• voluntary actions performed as part of physical activity and requiring varying amounts of energy dependent on the effort;
• growth, during the early years of life, in adolescence and during pregnancy.

Energy from food

All the energy required by the body must be supplied by food intake. The macronutrients in food and drink (carbohydrates, fats and proteins), together with alcohol, provide energy as they are broken down. The minerals and vitamins in food do not provide energy, although some are essential in the biochemical pathways that release energy.

Assumptions are made about the efficiency of digestion and absorption that may not be true in cases of illness involving diarrhoea or malabsorption syndromes, or when the diet contains large amounts of unabsorbable material, such as non-starch polysaccharides, or when laxatives are used.

Energy values of nutrients

The energy values used in the UK are:
Carbohydrates (as monosaccharides): 3.75 kcal/g (= 16 kJ/g)
Fat: 9 kcal/g (= 37 kJ/g)
Protein: 4 kcal/g (= 17 kJ/g)
Alcohol: 7 kcal/g (= 29 kJ/g)

Table 20.1 Example of use of energy conversion factors in calculation of energy content of foods.

Food	CHO (g/100 g)	Energy from CHO/100 g (A)	Fat (g/100 g)	Energy from fat/100 g (B)	Protein (g/100 g)	Energy from protein/100 g (C)	Total energy/100 g of food (A+B+C)
		Factor used: 3.75 kcal/g		*Factor used: 9 kcal/g*		*Factor used: 4 kcal/g*	
White bread	46.1	172.9	1.6	14.4	7.9	31.6	219
Milk, semi-skimmed	4.7	17.6	1.7	15.3	3.4	13.6	46
Baked beans	15.3	57.4	0.6	5.4	5.2	20.8	84

Calculation of the contribution of macronutrients to total energy intake

On the basis of the calculations illustrated in Table 20.1, it is also possible to calculate what percentage of the energy in a food is supplied by which macronutrient.

So, taking white bread:

$\frac{172.9}{219} \times 100 = 79\%$ of the energy comes from CHO

$\frac{31.6}{219} \times 100 = 14.4\%$ of the energy comes from protein, and

$\frac{14.4}{219} \times 100 = 6.6\%$ of the energy comes from fat.

Similar calculations could be performed for the other foods shown in Table 20.1; it can also be applied to a whole meal, or a day's intake of food.

Contribution of food groups to energy intake

The difficulty of obtaining accurate information about energy intakes from individuals is discussed in Chapter 3.

Information obtained from *household food surveys* in the UK provides an overview of the main contributors to the energy intake within the population; this is shown in Figure 20.1. It shows that:

• Cereals and cereals products are the main providers of energy, as they are in almost all countries in the world.

• A number of other food groups contribute similar amounts of energy to the overall intake.

• The majority of energy consumed (about 80%) is supplied by foods containing a range of nutrients; however, 10% comes from foods that contain only fat and 10% from foods containing only simple carbohydrate. These are foods that should be reduced if healthy eating guidelines are followed.

21 Energy intake: control

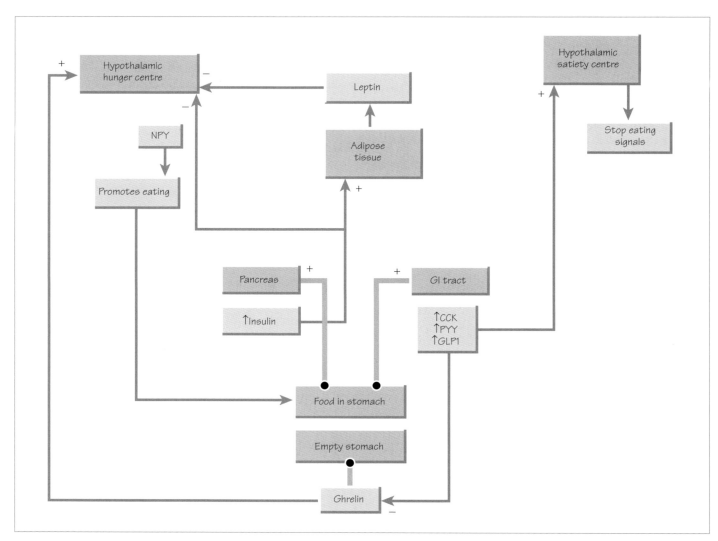

Fig. 21.1 Summary of physiological controls involved in eating.

Aims

(1) To investigate the physiological mechanisms that control food intake.

(2) To recognise the external influences on control of food intake.

Control of food intake

Food intake is necessary to satisfy the energy needs of the body, although energy stores provide a buffer against periods of starvation. Hunger and satiety are the sensations that indicate the need to start or stop eating – these represent the *physiological control* of eating.

Humans are exposed to many *external influences* that affect food intake, which may modify or over-ride the internal mechanisms.

Physiological control: internal mechanisms

A number of physiological mechanisms have been identified that regulate food intake to ensure energy supply, but avoid excessive storage. These mechanisms are believed to operate as a feedback system to meet energy needs.

Early work proposed that food intake was regulated by the need to control glucose, amino acid or temperature levels in the blood or to maintain a constant level of fat reserves. These mechanisms have not been totally discounted and probably play some role in short-term control of eating.

However, more recent work, mostly performed with animals, where feeding behaviour can be more readily controlled, has expanded this knowledge, to include a range of neurotransmitters, hormones and brain peptides that play a complex coordinating role in eating behaviour. Some of the factors appear to be involved in the drive to eat, others terminate eating. These are summarised in Figure 21.1.

Internal control signals

Ghrelin is a peptide hormone released from the endocrine cells of the stomach that signals hunger; on reaching the arcuate nucleus in the hypothalamus it stimulates the release of *neuropeptide Y* (NPY), which is a potent stimulant of food intake.

On eating, a number of *gut hormones* are released, including cholecystokinin (CCK), peptide YY (PYY 3–36) and glucagon-like peptide (GLP1). These hormones act both locally and centrally, to inhibit the release of ghrelin, slow down stomach emptying and stimulate hunger-reducing neurones in the hypothalamus.

The effects of these hormones are modulated by insulin and leptin.

- *Insulin* begins to be secreted from the pancreas within minutes of starting to eat. It is believed to potentiate the satiating effects of CCK.
- Insulin also has a central effect to reduce the size of the meal consumed.
- Insulin is involved in the secretion of *leptin* from adipose tissue, and eventually leptin inhibits insulin secretion.
- An increase in leptin levels inhibits NPY and therefore food intake.
- Insulin also inhibits NPY; fasting increases NPY synthesis, as insulin levels are low at this time.

Other neurotransmitter substances have been shown to have more specific association with particular dietary constituents. For example:

- *Serotonin* is released following consumption of carbohydrate, leading to a feeling of satisfaction. This may be linked to carbohydrate cravings.
- *Endorphins* (endogenous opiates) have been linked to the hedonic response to sugar and fat; blocking their release may reduce the desire for high-fat or sugary foods.

External influences

In humans, the importance of these fundamental physiological mechanisms is difficult to establish, as they appear to be readily over-ridden by the food environment and psychosocial factors.

Food is constantly available in most Western environments, so people make their choices on the basis of taste (palatability), cost, convenience and social trends.

- *Palatability* – for most consumers, especially the younger age groups, intake is associated with high-fat, high-sugar, high-salt foods, often developed to enhance their taste by the food industry. These foods have a high energy density. It is only as people become older that there appears to be a change to a less energy-dense diet.
- *Cost* – foods containing higher levels of fat and sugar are often cheaper than more nutrient-dense items. In addition, there has been a move towards selling foods in larger portion sizes, which appear financially economical. When there are financial constraints, the consumer looks for maximum dietary energy for minimum cost and hence is more likely to choose the higher fat/sugary foods.
- *Convenience* – the perceived busy lifestyle of many people has led to a desire for readily available food that is easily consumed with minimum preparation needed. The response of the food industry has been to produce an enormous range of prepared meals and fast foods that fulfil these requirements. Diets based on fast or ready prepared foods have been found to have energy density up to 60% greater than a more traditional British diet.
- *Snacking* – associated with the search for convenience is the move away from a 'three-meal-a-day' tradition, and a pattern of eating that may include a much greater number of snacks during the day, of which none may be nutrient rich, but all of which may have a high energy density. In addition, soft drinks with a high energy density are believed to contribute energy, but have no satiety effect.
- *Social and peer pressure* – eating is a social activity, maintained and constrained by cultural factors. This can modify individual physiological eating controls, by the need to comply with peer pressure, e.g. to eat fast food, snack, control body weight by restrained eating or following a particular diet plan, develop (positive or negative) attitudes to specific foods and even take exercise to increase physical activity. All of these make it very difficult for an individual to respond to their own food needs being signalled by the physiological control mechanisms.

Summary

Food intake is essential for survival, and there are physiological mechanisms to regulate it. The environmental factors encountered by many consumers result in poor regulation of food intake and consequently excessive consumption of energy in relation to needs.

All of these factors make it very challenging for public health policy-makers to address the rising incidence of overweight in most societies.

Aims

(1) To consider the ways in which energy needs can be measured.

Even when at complete rest, the human body uses energy in maintaining a range of physiological functions. Energy usage increases when:

- food needs to be digested;
- there is any additional movement;
- body temperature needs to be increased.

Energy therefore needs to be supplied at all times, either from food intake or stored reserves. This represents the body's *need for energy*, or the *energy requirement*.

Principles of energy use

Energy is supplied from the combustion or oxidation of the macronutrients from food, in a controlled fashion, via a number of biochemical pathways. The energy released is used mainly to synthesise ATP from ADP and inorganic phosphate. During periods of fasting, energy stores are mobilised, by the action of hormones (including glucagon, growth hormone and cortisol), and oxidised to maintain the energy supply.

Both the synthesis and utilisation of ATP (in biosynthesis, maintenance of electrical cellular gradients and mechanical work) are energetically inefficient processes, with heat being a major byproduct.

Measurement of energy expenditure

Direct calorimetry

Measurement of heat output is an indicator of the energy transformations occurring in the body, and is the basis of direct calorimetry as a means of obtaining values for energy output. In practice this can be performed in a metabolic chamber, a room where the subject can live; the heat output of the subject is detected by sensors in the walls of the room. This equates to the energy expenditure. The physical limitations of this environment make it a less than practical method, but measurements made in this way have enabled other methods to be developed.

Indirect calorimetry

A more practical approach is to utilise the information about gas exchanges that occur during metabolic reactions, and the associated heat/energy output. These can be predicted from chemical formulae of the substrates and metabolic equations.

The stoichiometric equation for the oxidation of glucose is given below; similar equations exist showing the oxidation of other substrates:

$$C_6H_{12}O_6 + 6O_2 = 6H_2O + 6CO_2 + 15.5\,kJ/g \text{ of energy}$$

$$(180\,g) + (6 \times 22.4\,L) = (6 \times 18\,g) + (6 \times 22.4\,L) + (2.78\,MJ)$$

From the above it can be calculated that in glucose oxidation, for each litre of oxygen consumed, the heat output is 20.7 kJ (this is based on the release of 2780 kJ when 6×22.4 litres of oxygen are consumed). Similar calculations can be performed to obtain heat output per litre of oxygen, for the oxidation of alcohol, fats and proteins (these are shown in Table 22.1).

Therefore if the amount of oxygen consumed can be measured, this would allow the calculation of the amount of heat produced or energy expended.

Greater accuracy can be introduced into the calculation of energy output by measuring urinary nitrogen, which allows incomplete metabolism of amino acids to be taken into account.

Various methods of obtaining information about *gas exchanges* exist. In principle gases must be collected and analysed over a period of time. This can be achieved in:

- a closed system, such as a collecting bag (e.g. Douglas bag);
- a system where the flow of gases is continuously analysed, such as a ventilated hood, tent or canopy, which can also be attached to other respiratory equipment in the clinical setting.

Interference with normal respiratory patterns is a major obstacle and care must be taken to allow a period of equilibration. Fixed equipment limits the range of activities that can be studied.

The introduction of the *doubly-labelled water* (DLW) technique has provided a means of obtaining energy output data from free-living

Respiratory quotient (RQ)

The stoichiometric equations show the amount of carbon dioxide produced and oxygen consumed for a given amount of each substrate. This ratio (CO_2:O_2) is known as the respiratory quotient (RQ).

- If both oxygen consumption and carbon dioxide output are measured over a period of time, the RQ can be determined and the energy equivalent at the given RQ of oxygen consumed is computed.
- RQ varies with the substrate being metabolised; in practice, over a period of 24 hours, one can expect that the mixture of macronutrients used reflects their balance in a typical diet. Thus for a Western diet with 35% fat and 15% protein, the RQ would be 0.87. This can be confirmed from concurrently kept dietary records.
- Similarly, the energy yield per litre of oxygen is also rounded to a mean of 20.3 kJ/L when details about RQ are not available.

Table 22.1 Heat output per litre of oxygen consumed for different metabolic substrates.

Nutrient	Oxygen consumed (L/g)	Carbon dioxide produced (L/g)	RQ	Energy equivalent (kJ/L of O_2)
Glucose	0.746	0.746	1.0	20.7
Fats (mean)	1.975	1.402	0.71	19.8
Protein	0.962	0.775	0.81	19.25
Alcohol	1.429	0.966	0.663	20.4

Doubly-labelled water (DLW) technique

(1) Subject drinks a small amount of 'heavy' water, labelled with deuterium and oxygen-18 (^2H_2O and $H_2^{18}O$). These are naturally occurring nonradioactive isotopes of water.

(2) The hydrogen equilibrates with the body water, and is washed out as part of body water turnover.

(3) The oxygen-18 is also lost with body water, but in addition is incorporated into carbon dioxide and lost in this way. Thus oxygen-18 is lost faster than deuterium.

(4) Samples of urine are collected over a period of up to 14 days and the rate of loss of the isotopes monitored. The difference between these represents the carbon dioxide turnover.

subjects in a noninvasive and nonintrusive manner. Measurements can be collected for periods of 7–14 days, in various situations and in subjects of all ages. The method has become the 'gold standard' against which other methods are compared. Unfortunately, the costs and availability of the labelled water make this unsuitable for large-scale studies.

Noncalorimetric methods

The use of heart rate monitoring, or motion sensors can provide information about physical activity. However, the validity of these techniques for accurate estimation of energy needs has not been determined.

Equations for metabolic rate

In practice, experimental methods for obtaining a measure of basal metabolic rate (BMR; or resting metabolic rate, RMR) may not be feasible. A number of equations have been developed, based on measurements of large numbers of subjects, that allow BMR to be calculated, given a number of key indicators about the subjects, including age, gender and body weight.

Those most commonly used are the Schofield and Harris–Benedict equations. Although the latter were developed from limited data in the early 1900s, they are still in widespread use, especially in the USA. Schofield equations for calculating BMR are shown in Table 22.2.

Table 22.2 Formulae for calculating BMR (MJ/day) (Schofield equations).

	Age range (years)	Regression formula for BMR (MJ/day)
Men	10–17	$0.074 \times$ weight (kg) + 2.754
	18–29	$0.063 \times$ weight (kg) + 2.896
	30–59	$0.048 \times$ weight (kg) + 3.653
	60–74	$0.0499 \times$ weight (kg) + 2.930
	75+	$0.0350 \times$ weight (kg) + 3.434
Women	10–17	$0.056 \times$ weight (kg) + 3.434
	18–29	$0.062 \times$ weight (kg) + 2.036
	30–59	$0.034 \times$ weight (kg) + 3.538
	60–74	$0.0386 \times$ weight (kg) + 2.875
	75+	$0.0410 \times$ weight (kg) + 2.610

23 Energy requirements: components

Aims

(1) To identify the components of energy output.
(2) To explore the determinants of energy output and requirements.

Components of energy expenditure

Three main components are generally identified:

- basal (or resting) metabolic rate;
- thermic effect of food;
- physical activity.

In addition, growth during the very early periods of life increases energy expenditure.

Basal metabolic rate (BMR)

This is the energy expended by the body in:

- maintaining active transport across cellular membranes;
- contraction of fibres in mechanical work (such as respiration and heartbeat);
- synthesis of new molecules.

The concept of BMR does not include any internal processing of food or muscular effort. Therefore measurement of BMR is performed under strict conditions:

- fasting;
- mental and physical relaxation;
- at a comfortable environmental temperature.

For practical purposes, resting metabolic rate (RMR) is used, which allows a more realistic baseline measurement. It is estimated to be approximately 3% higher over 24 hours than BMR. However, these terms tend to be used interchangeably.

An average value for an adult male is approximately 4.2 kJ (1 kcal)/min, and remains relatively constant. There is, however, variation between individuals, attributable to the factors described in the Box below.

For most sedentary individuals, the BMR accounts for 60–70% of the daily energy expenditure.

Thermic effect of food (TEF)

This is also known as diet-induced thermogenesis or obligatory thermogenesis, and represents the stimulation of metabolism as a result of the processing of food and storage of macronutrients. It lasts for 3–6 hours, and is estimated to be equivalent to 10% of the energy content of the meal (or 10% of the total energy output for 24 hours). TEF is greater with protein- and carbohydrate-containing meals than with fats.

Physical activity

This is the *most variable component* of daily energy expenditure, but the one over which individuals have most control. The amount of energy expended during any type of physical activity is related to the body size, and through this, to the BMR.

Adaptive thermogenesis

Research indicates that in certain individuals there exists a capacity for adaptive thermogenesis, which allows the body to dissipate excess energy intake as heat, using futile cycles that do not generate ATP.

This has been shown to be associated with uncoupling proteins (UCP), some of the genes for which have been identified. Varying levels of UCP activity in brown adipose tissue (BAT) have been demonstrated in animals that could resist weight gain consequent on overfeeding.

The importance of these mechanisms in humans remains unclear. It has been proposed that this was a mechanism of evolutionary advantage when nutrient-poor diets had to be consumed in large amounts, providing large amounts of energy with little nutritional content. The ability to dissipate the excessive energy allowed individuals to extract nutrients without becoming overweight. The prevalence of adequate food supplies makes this unnecessary in present times.

Major determinants of BMR

- **Weight:** Energy output is determined by cell mass, therefore body weight is a key determinant of BMR. Heavier individuals thus have a higher BMR.
- **Gender:** BMR is related to muscle mass, which is greater in males than females, resulting in a higher BMR for the same body weight. Women have a higher proportion of body fat, which has a lower BMR/kg than muscle.
- **Age:** BMR, expressed per kg body weight, declines from infancy to old age, as the active cell mass decreases. The increment for growth is relatively small, averaging 21 kJ (5 kcal)/g of tissue gained. The additional requirement for growth is therefore greatest at periods of growth spurts (in the first months of life, at the peak of puberty).
- **Genetic factors:** There are differences in metabolic rate between people, but these have yet to be fully investigated. They probably account for less than 10% of the variability in BMR between individuals.
- **Other factors:** These include certain drugs and pharmacological agents (nicotine, caffeine, amphetamines, capsaicin in chillies), disease states (fever, thyroid disease, cancers) and environmental conditions (extreme heat or cold). Fasting may result in a reduction in BMR, as the body attempts to adapt to a perceived life-threatening situation (even if this is brought about consciously by the individual in an attempt to lose weight).

Therefore the amount of energy expended in activity is described in terms of factors, known as *physical activity ratios* (PARs), which indicate the ratio by which energy output is raised above the resting (BMR) value. Values have been published by the UK's Department of Health (1991) (see Appendix 3).

These ratios have been derived from many measurements of a wide range of activities, and can be used to calculate the incremental energy expended during a period of time from records of the activities undertaken. These figures are averages and do not accurately quantify the intensity of the activity or the amount of effort exerted. They should be used with caution in making judgements about energy ouput.

When intense physical activity is undertaken, there is a residual effect on the BMR, which persists for several hours and up to 24 hours with severe exercise. It is believed that this is associated with repair and recovery processes occurring in muscles.

Non-exercise activity related thermogenesis (NEAT) is an additional component of energy output that describes the small-scale movements that can be collectively described as 'fidgeting'. Although these appear to be minimal, their continuation throughout long periods of time suggests that they may account for substantial amounts of energy expenditure and may explain the ability of some individuals to maintain a normal weight.

Calculating total energy expenditure (TEE)

This is generally done from records of 24-hour periods of activity, and using formulae for BMR and PAR values. An example is given in Table 23.1.

TEF is generally not included separately in these calculations, as it is considered to be subsumed within the PAR for eating.

Thus Joe expended 11.07 MJ during the course of the day. As his BMR is 7.01 MJ, it is possible to calculate his overall physical activity level (PAL) for the day, that is, the ratio by which his

Table 23.1 Example calculation of energy expenditure. Joe kept a record of his activities during one day. He is 45 years old and weighs 70 kg. His BMR is therefore $(0.048 \times 70) + 3.653 = 7.01$ MJ/day, or $(7010/24)$ kJ/h = 292 kJ/h.

Activity	Duration (h)	PAR	BMR/h	Energy used (kJ)
Duration × PAR × BMR = Energy used				
Sleeping	6	1.0	292	1752
Personal activities (washing, dressing, eating)	2	1.4	292	818
Driving to and from work	2	2.0	292	1168
Sitting at work (light office work)	9	1.5	292	3942
Cycle ride	2	4.0	292	2336
Watching TV	3	1.2	292	1051
Total for the day	24			11 067

energy output was increased above BMR for the whole day. This is $(11.07/7.01) = 1.58$. Overall he used almost 60% more energy than his BMR.

Compared with the typical population, whose PAL averages 1.4, Joe was relatively active. This probably arises from his moderate activity at work and the cycle ride after work.

Summary

Overall energy expenditure is largely dependent on body size, which determines the basal metabolic rate, as well as the amount of energy used in physical activities. However, it is physical activity that has the greatest impact on daily energy output. Even relatively small increments in activity can make a difference to daily output, and people are encouraged to include these in daily routines, to maintain energy balance.

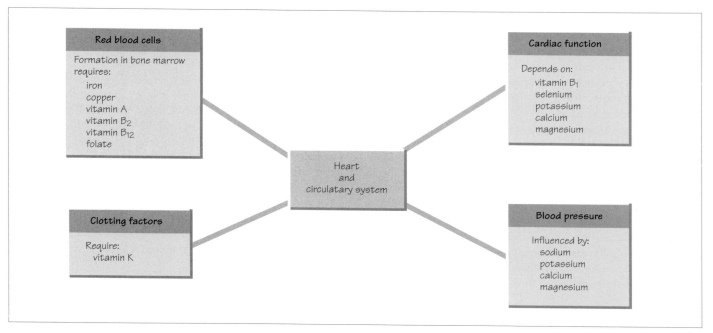

Fig. 24.1 Overview of micronutrients that interact to support the heart and circulatory system.

Aims

(1) To consider the micronutrients of importance in maintaining cardiac function.
(2) To identify the micronutrients that may affect blood pressure.
(3) To consider how blood clotting is affected by levels of micronutrients.

A number of micronutrients interact to maintain the heart and circulatory system, including the production of the formed elements of the blood. Figure 24.1 gives an overview.

Cardiac function

In maintaining the circulation, the cardiac muscle must be supplied with adequate nutrition to sustain its function. In addition to the normal macronutrients needed for energy supply, the heart is especially vulnerable to deficiencies in certain micronutrients.

Thiamin is involved in the release of energy in biochemical reactions. Deficiency signs include cardiac enlargement and oedema, associated with increased levels of pyruvate and lactate in the blood, causing vasodilation and increased workload for the heart. Thiamin may improve cardiac function also in patients with chronic heart failure.

Selenium acts as an antioxidant, and a deficiency has been associated with a cardiomyopathy, which in severe cases is associated with multiple necrosis throughout the heart muscle; this is, however, rare.

Plasma **potassium**, **calcium** and **magnesium** levels must all be kept within strict limits for the normal electrical activity of the heart. Abnormal levels, which can result in arrhythmias, are likely to reflect pathological processes, or the effects of drug action, rather than dietary inadequacies.

Blood pressure

Sodium is the main cation found in the blood and extracellular fluid, where it accounts for 95% of the cations. As such it plays a major role in the regulation of body fluids, including blood pressure and acid–base balance.

The control of plasma sodium levels depends on a balance between sodium excretion and absorption at the kidneys, regulated by neural and hormonal mechanisms, including renin, angiotensin and aldosterone, which regulate sodium levels, and antidiuretic hormone and atrial natriuretic peptide, which balance the water levels in response.

Changes in sodium levels can affect blood pressure, but are not in themselves necessarily the cause of high blood pressure. Nevertheless, there is considerable evidence to support the proposition that reducing sodium intakes can effect a reduction in blood pressure (see Chapter 58).

Potassium is predominantly an intracellular ion and is associated in exchange mechanisms with sodium. Increased dietary intakes of potassium have been associated with reduction in blood pressure, as it promotes natriuresis (loss of sodium in the urine). It is proposed that an increase in potassium intakes to offset some of the sodium in the diet would be beneficial for cardiovascular health.

Sodium intakes
Sodium is mainly consumed as an ingredient of processed foods, including meat products, cereal products, cheese and snack foods. Sodium intakes from natural sources would be only 10% of those currently consumed.

Calcium is also important in blood pressure regulation, and diets rich in calcium, especially from dairy products, have been found to be effective in reducing blood pressure.

Normal **magnesium** levels maintain smooth muscle tone, and are implicated in control of blood pressure. Magnesium may also protect cardiac muscle from injury during ischaemia.

Studies on pre-eclampsia in pregnant women have found a beneficial effect of magnesium supplementation to prevent the elevation of blood pressure. Food sources of magnesium include whole-grain cereals, nuts, legumes and green leafy vegetables.

Clotting factors

Four of the factors involved in the clotting cascade contain γ-carboxyglutamates; these are prothrombin and factors VII, IX and X.

Vitamin K acts as an essential cofactor in the gamma carboxylation of glutamic acid, and is therefore required for the synthesis of the clotting factors. Deficiency of vitamin K, or interference with its metabolic role, has a major impact on blood clotting.

Warfarin, which is extensively used as an anticoagulant drug, prevents the regeneration of vitamin K and interferes with this reaction.

Dietary deficiency of vitamin K is rare because the vitamin is widespread, although the richest sources are dark-green vegetables and vegetable oils and spreads (including products containing these).

The vitamin is also synthesised in the colon by bacteria, but there are situations in which this synthesis is inhibited, such as prolonged antibiotic therapy, use of mineral oil laxatives and in fat malabsorption syndromes.

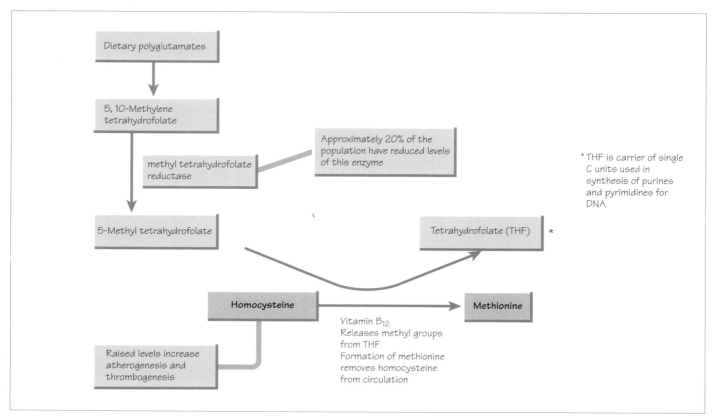

Fig. 25.2 Interaction between folate and vitamin B_{12} in formation of DNA and regulation of homocysteine levels.

Aims

(1) To identify and describe the micronutrients of importance in the formation and function of red blood cells.

Red blood cells (RBCs)

RBCs transport oxygen from the lungs to the tissues and also carbon dioxide to the lungs. Oxygen transport occurs by incorporation into haemoglobin, which is a ferrous iron-containing molecule. Therefore **iron** is critical in the function of RBCs.

Iron in the body

Approximately 60% of the body's iron content (total ~4 g) is found in haemoglobin and 15% in the bone marrow, where RBC production occurs. The remainder is:
• stored as ferritin in liver, bone marrow and spleen; ferritin is a protein containing up to 4000 atoms of iron in its interior to minimise toxic effects; plasma ferritin levels reflect iron stores;
• in functional enzymes (such as cytochromes) throughout cells;
• in myoglobin in muscle (a pigment with a high affinity for oxygen);
• in small amounts in the circulation, attached to transferrin, the iron-transport protein.

Iron intake and absorption

Two forms of iron occur in the diet: haem (organic) and non-haem (inorganic). Sources of haem iron include meat, liver, fish and eggs.

Sources of non-haem iron include cereals (breakfast cereals and white bread are fortified in the UK), legumes, green vegetables, nuts, dried fruit and chocolate.

The absorption of haem iron is greater than that of non-haem iron. The latter is very susceptible to promoting and inhibiting factors (see Table 25.1), which can make a tenfold difference to the efficiency of absorption. Advising people to enhance promoting factors and reduce inhibitors can make a substantial difference to iron status.

Table 25.1 Factors affecting absorption of non-haem iron.

Factors promoting absorption	Factors inhibiting absorption
Vitamin C	Phytate (in whole cereal grains)
Citric acid	Polyphenols (in tea, coffee and nuts)
Lactic acid	Oxalic acid (in tea, spinach)
Fructose	Phosphates (in egg yolk)
Peptides from protein sources, especially meat	Calcium
	Zinc
These enhance the solubility of the iron, facilitating absorption	*These either bind with iron, making it less soluble, or compete for binding sites*

Iron absorption is tightly controlled to match the body's need, as iron is toxic to cells because of its pro-oxidant properties. Ingested iron not immediately required remains in the enterocytes, and is shed at the end of their life cycle in the faeces.

There is no capacity for excretion of absorbed iron, other than by loss of blood or shedding of cells.

Breakdown of RBCs in the reticuloendothelial system provides the endogenous source of iron. Up to 25–30 mg of iron is transported in the body per day from sites of absorption or release for storage or utilisation.

Iron deficiency anaemia (IDA) is the most common nutritional deficiency in the world, with a range of pathological consequences. These can include changes to the digestive tract, loss of appetite, reduced work capacity and eventually heart failure.

IDA can also affect the function of white blood cells, reducing their ability to destroy invading organisms.

Addressing IDA involves a number of measures, including:
- fortification of widely consumed foods;
- use of supplements;
- education to improve dietary practices to enhance bioavailability of iron consumed;
- introduction of greater diversity of iron sources into the diet.

Other nutrients affecting RBCs

Copper is also found in RBCs, and in plasma as caeruloplasmin. This converts ferrous iron to the ferric form, which binds to transferrin, for carriage to synthesis or storage sites. Copper deficiency can result in hypochromic anaemia. Dietary copper deficiency is rare in humans, although there is a rare congenital condition, Menke's disease, which affects copper absorption.

Vitamin A facilitates the use of storage iron for haemopoiesis, and IDA can be a consequence of vitamin A deficiency.

Deficiency of **riboflavin** can result in hypochromic anaemia as a result of impaired iron absorption. **Pyridoxine** (vitamin B_6) is utilised in the incorporation of iron into haem, and thus has a role in RBC formation.

Folate and vitamin B_{12} are used in the formation of purines and pyrimidines for the synthesis of DNA and RNA and as such are crucial for cell division.
- Folate (as tetrahydrofolate, THF) carries single-carbon units (e.g. methyl groups), derived from amino acids such as serine and glycine, which are used in this biosynthesis.
- Vitamin B_{12} is required to release the single carbon units and regenerate THF to enable it to receive further single carbon units. This is termed the 'methyl trap', and without B_{12}, the methylation of DNA may become inadequate to sustain gene transcription.
- The methyl group removed during this reaction is used in the formation of methionine from homocysteine, and helps to lower plasma homocysteine levels (see Figure 25.2). Elevated homocysteine may be a contributory factor in atherosclerosis (see Chapter 57).
- Both folate and B_{12} deficiencies result in an inability of developing cells to increase their DNA prior to division. RBCs are therefore large (megaloblastic), have a reduced density and are fewer in number; this results in reduced oxygen-carrying capacity of the blood, and anaemia.

Overall, the nutrients involved in maintaining the blood and circulatory system can be obtained from a varied diet, in line with healthy eating recommendations (Table 25.2).

Table 25.2 A summary of the nutrients required by the blood and circulatory system, and their sources in a balanced diet.

Food groups in healthy eating recommendations	Nutrients supplied relevant to blood and circulation
Bread, cereals, starchy foods and potatoes (whole grain products preferred)	Iron, magnesium, potassium Thiamin
Fruit and vegetables	Iron, copper, magnesium, potassium Folate, vitamin A, vitamin K
Meat, fish and alternatives (including pulses, nuts and seeds)	Iron, copper, sodium, potassium Vitamin B_{12}, vitamin A
Milk and dairy products	Sodium, calcium Vitamin B_{12}, riboflavin
Fatty and sugary foods	Vitamin K, sodium

26 Micronutrients: role in metabolism

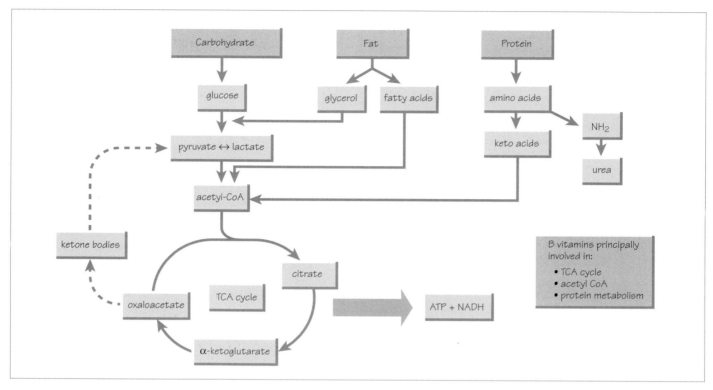

Fig. 26.1 Overview of the link between macronutrient metabolism and TCA cycle, and role of B vitamins.

Aims

(1) To identify the micronutrients involved in energy-producing metabolic pathways.
(2) To consider other roles of these micronutrients and any interactions between them.

Overview of metabolism

Central to metabolism is the tricarboxylic acid (TCA) cycle; products from all three macronutrients ultimately enter this pathway (Figure 26.1).

Energy release in metabolic pathways occurs as a result of oxidation; removal of hydrogen atoms and their transfer to hydrogen acceptor molecules is a common step. Acceptor molecules form the *electron transport chain* in oxidative phosphorylation, producing ATP, and ultimately carbon dioxide and water. Acceptor molecules are nicotinamide adenine dinucleotide (NAD), flavin mononucleotide (FMN), flavin adenine dinucleotide (FAD) and cytochromes.

The *B group of vitamins act as cofactors in metabolism* (Table 26.1). In general they:

- facilitate the release of energy;
- are involved in the electron transport chain;
- act as cofactors in the synthesis of metabolic derivatives.

Thiamin (vitamin B_1) is used in its active form, thiamin diphosphate (or thiamin pyrophosphate, TPP). Thiamin diphosphate has

Table 26.1 Principal roles of B vitamins in metabolism.

Vitamin	CHO	Fats	Proteins	Other
Thiamin	✓			
Riboflavin	✓	✓	✓	Purine catabolism
				Neurotransmitter synthesis
				Antioxidant role
				Metabolism of other minerals/vitamins
Niacin	✓	✓	✓	Steroid hormone synthesis
				Cholesterol synthesis
Vitamin B_6	✓		✓	Steroid hormone activity
Pantothenic acid	✓	✓	✓	Acetylcholine synthesis
				Joint structure and lubrication
Biotin	✓	✓		Gluconeogenesis, fatty acid synthesis

a central role in the TCA cycle and carbohydrate metabolism, as a cofactor for:

- pyruvate dehydrogenase: whereby acetyl coenzyme A is produced from pyruvate at the start of the TCA cycle;
- α-ketoglutarate dehydrogenase, within the TCA cycle;
- branched-chain keto acid dehydrogenase, which completes the metabolism of valine, leucine and isoleucine, whose products can also enter the TCA cycle;
- transketolase in the pentose phosphate pathway, which metabolises glucose, is a source of reduced nicotinamide adenine dinucleotide

phosphate (NADPH) for fatty acid synthesis, and five-carbon sugars for DNA synthesis.

Riboflavin (vitamin B_2) forms a part of two flavin coenzymes:

- flavin mononucleotide (FMN);
- flavin adenine dinucleotide (FAD).

The flavin coenzymes play a role in:

- fatty acid oxidation;
- purine catabolism (with xanthine oxidase);
- neurotransmitter synthesis (with monoamine oxidases);
- drug metabolism (with mixed function oxidases);
- glutathione reductase (an antioxidant role, in conjunction with selenium).

In addition, riboflavin interacts with other nutrients in the metabolism of folate, pyridoxine and vitamin A, conversion of tryptophan to niacin, and iron absorption from the digestive tract.

Riboflavin is very efficiently recycled in the body, so that deficiency is not fatal; marginal deficiency appears to be relatively widespread. Needs are increased during growth and tissue repair, and turnover is higher in catabolic states.

Pathological changes associated with deficiency affect:

- the mouth – lesions to the lips (cheilosis), corners of the mouth (angular stomatitis) and the tongue (glossitis);
- the eyes – conjunctivitis, photosensitivity and vascularisation of the cornea;
- the skin – affected by dermatitis, especially of the nose, cheeks and forehead.

Niacin is the generic name for nicotinic acid and nicotinamide, used to form nicotinamide adenine dinucleotide (NAD) and NAD phosphate (NADP).

Nicotinamide can be synthesised in the body from tryptophan (requires riboflavin and vitamin B_6) and despite a low conversion rate (generally 60:1) this is sufficient in Western diets to meet the needs for niacin. A dietary source of niacin becomes essential only in low-protein diets.

NAD mainly acts as a *hydrogen acceptor in oxidative reactions*, forming NADH (needed for gluconeogenesis), in:

- energy-yielding reactions, such as glycolysis;
- the TCA cycle;
- β-oxidation of fatty acids;
- oxidation of alcohol.

NADP is mainly used as NADPH (generated by the pentose phosphate pathway), in energy-requiring reactions such as synthesis of fatty acids, glutamate and cholesterol.

Vitamin B_6 is the collective name given to pyridoxine, pyridoxal and pyridoxamine, which are interconverted within the body; the active form of the vitamin is pyridoxal phosphate (PLP).

The main metabolic roles are:

- *Amino acid metabolism:* over 100 enzymes use PLP as a coenzyme. Reactions include transamination, deamination, decarboxylation and transulphuration.
- *Glycogen phosphorylation:* the release of glucose from stored glycogen requires PLP as a coenzyme; the majority of PLP is found in muscle associated with this enzyme.
- *Regulation of steroid hormone activity:* PLP terminates the action of steroid hormones on the nuclear receptor.

Pantothenic acid is a part of the coenzyme A molecule, and therefore central to metabolism. It plays a part in the TCA cycle, oxidation of carbohydrates and ketogenic amino acids, and synthesis of fatty acids. Coenzyme A is involved in the synthesis of acetylcholine, cholesterol, hyaluronic acid and chondroitin sulphate found in joints.

Biotin has a widespread role, as a cofactor for carboxylase enzymes, which carry carbon dioxide units in many metabolic pathways. These include gluconeogenesis (which requires pyruvate carboxylase) and fatty acid synthesis (using acetyl CoA carboxylase).

27 Micronutrients: protective and defence roles I

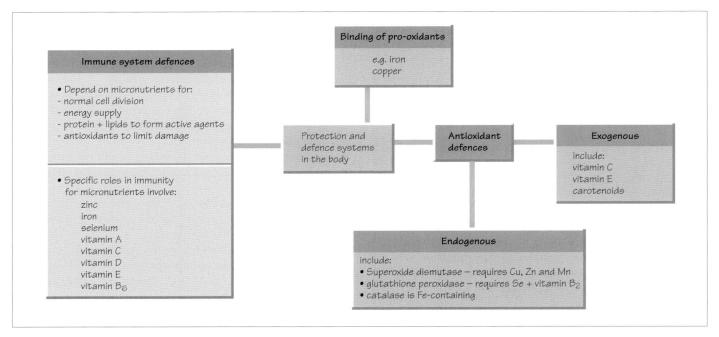

Fig. 27.1 Overview of protective and defence systems and micronutrient involvement.

Aims

(1) To identify the nutrients involved in sustaining the functions of the immune system.

Physiological systems are continually challenged by changes in the *internal* environment from metabolic or defence reactions and also by *external* factors, such as microorganisms, or chemical substances that enter the body.

Various systems or mechanisms exist to maintain homeostasis. An overview is given in Figure 27.1, which shows that the majority of these defence mechanisms depend on micronutrients for their operation.

Inadequate levels of some micronutrients can compromise this protection and increase the risk of diseases; conversely, adequate or enhanced levels may be actively protective.

Immune system defences

The immune system plays a crucial role in protecting the body against the dangers posed by infection, inflammation and trauma. The cells of the immune system and their products require an appropriate nutrient supply to produce these components and sustain them.

• Formation of the cellular components requires normal cell division to be sustained.

• Macronutrients are needed to provide the energy for the metabolic activity of the cells; in conjunction with these, many micronutrients are needed to release this energy (see Chapter 26).

• When the immune system is responding to a challenge, energy requirements are increased.

• The immune defence includes a number of proteins (immuno-globulins, cytokines, acute-phase proteins) and lipid-derived substances (such as prostaglandins), which are synthesised from the appropriate amino acid and lipid precursors.

• Invading organisms are killed by an oxidative burst, which uses superoxide radicals, and can result in oxidative damage to the host cells. Appropriate antioxidant mechanisms must be in place as protection against this.

Nutritional inadequacy compromises the immune system and its ability to respond. This is seen in malnourished individuals, especially children, who are exceptionally vulnerable to infections, and are unable to recover swiftly from them. The condition is aggravated by a loss of appetite, possible malabsorption, increased loss of nutrients and higher requirements.

Specific micronutrients can be shown to play particular roles in the immune system. It should not, however, be assumed that high levels of these nutrients are necessarily ideal, as in some cases they may have a detrimental effect.

Vitamin A is important for:
• integrity of epidermal and mucosal surfaces, and thus the physical barrier against the environment;
• activation of macrophages and differentiation of monocytes in the immune response.

Deficiency is associated with increased incidence and severity of infectious diseases, especially respiratory and diarrhoeal diseases and measles; supplementation with vitamin A significantly reduces mortality from infection. However, very high doses of vitamin A can depress immune function. In many developing countries, vitamin A intake is low, and single large doses of the vitamin can be given as a supplement to help protect children from infection.

Table 27.1 Summary of principal micronutrients involved in the maintenance of the immune system.

Nutrient	Role in immune system	Evidence of importance
Vitamin A	Maintains epithelial surface; physical barrier Activates macrophages	Deficiency associated with incidence and severity of infectious disease
Vitamin B_6	DNA and RNA formation for lymphocytes and cytokine production	Impaired immune response in older subjects, reversed on supplementation
Vitamin C	Concentrated in white blood cells, as antioxidant protects against free radical damage of phagocytosis	May reduce severity of cold symptoms
Vitamin D	Present in immune cells, may be immunosuppressive	
Vitamin E	Enhances humoral and cellular immunity	Supplementation improves immune responses in older adults
Zinc	Development of T-lymphocytes Activity of immune cells	Effectively used in treatment for diarrhoea associated with poor nutrition
Iron	Low status inhibits phagocytic activity Improved status may encourage pathogen growth	
Selenium	Deficiency associated with reduced ability to kill pathogens	

Vitamin B_6 is used in the synthesis of nucleic acids for DNA and RNA formation. Impairment of this process affects lymphocyte proliferation and cytokine production and hence impacts on immune function in deficiency states. Supplementation reverses this impairment.

Although both **folate** and **vitamin B_{12}** are also involved in the synthesis of DNA and RNA, their effects on the function of the immune system are less obvious than might be expected.

Vitamin C concentration in leucocytes is high, and decreases during the course of an infection, due to dilution by newly released cells with lower vitamin content. Neutrophils contain high levels of vitamin C to protect against the oxidative burst.

However, excessively high intakes of vitamin C (>600 mg/day) can inhibit the formation of superoxide and reduce the effectiveness of neutrophils.

There are receptors for **vitamin D** in most immune cells, implying a regulatory role; most evidence suggests an immunosuppressant role, although further work is needed.

Supplementation with **vitamin E** enhances both humoral and cellular immunity, possibly by reducing the potential immunosuppressive effects of free radicals and lipid peroxides. However, doses above 800 mg/day may be counterproductive.

Zinc is important for the development of many of the cellular components of the immune system, especially the T-lymphocytes, and the activity of the cells. This includes chemotaxis, phagocytic activity and the oxidative burst. There is a fall in plasma zinc levels on infection, which may deprive the pathogens of essential zinc, and is an important protective response against potential pro-oxidant effects. Zinc is taken up at this time by the liver and lymphocytes.

Zinc supplementation at an appropriate dose has been found to be an effective treatment in diarrhoea associated with poor nutrition.

Vitamin C vs the common cold?

The balance of evidence in relation to vitamin C giving protection against the common cold points to a reduced severity of symptoms, but no reduction in the risk of infection.

Dietary zinc

Zinc in the diet tends to accompany protein, so low-protein diets are likely to be low in zinc. Good sources are lean meat, seafoods and dairy products.

Pulses and whole-grain cereals are important for non-meat-eaters.

Absorption of zinc is affected by promoters (animal products, amino acids) and inhibitors (binding to insoluble salts, such as phytate, phosphate, and the presence of large amounts of iron or calcium in the diet).

Decreased lymphocyte numbers are also a feature of **copper** deficiency, reversible on repletion. Excess amounts of copper have an immunosuppressive effect.

The role of **iron** in the immune system is complex. Low iron status impairs the ability of neutrophils to kill pathogens, and proliferation of lymphocytes.

Treatment of iron-deficient individuals is frequently associated with an exacerbation of infection; possibly the result of enhancement of growth of the pathogen by the additional iron.

Selenium deficiency is associated with reduced immunocompetence, in particular the ability of cells to kill pathogens. In tissues that are experiencing oxidative stress, due to impaired antioxidant status, viruses may mutate to more virulent forms. This has been proposed in selenium deficiency, but may be exacerbated by concurrent vitamin E deficiency and excess intakes of polyunsaturated fats.

This demonstrates the importance of an adequate level of a range of micronutrients to support normal immune function.

The question of supplementation with micronutrients remains unresolved, as high levels of some may be counterproductive, suppressing immune function. In addition, an imbalance may increase the requirements for other components. A balanced diet, following healthy eating guidelines, is the better alternative. It also provides phytochemicals, which may have important, as yet unrecognised, roles.

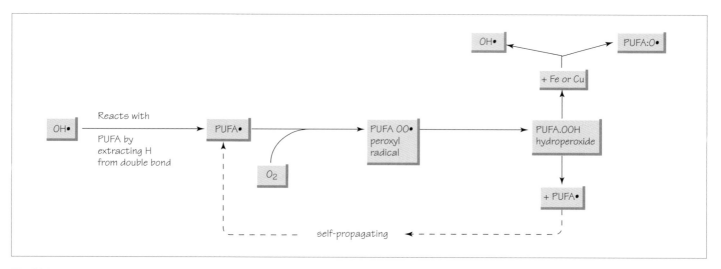

Fig. 28.1 Example of free radical-induced chain reaction in polyunsaturated fatty acid (e.g. in cell membrane).

Aims

(1) To explain the potential risks from free radicals in the body.
(2) To consider the role of micronutrients in antioxidant defence systems.

Free radicals

Free radicals and oxygen-derived radicals (also known as reactive oxygen species, ROS), are considered to be particularly harmful in the body.

These are highly reactive species that contain one or more unpaired electrons, which makes them unstable. They are produced when a covalent bond is broken, or by the gain or loss of a single electron.

Examples include the hydrogen radical ($H^{\bullet}$), hydroxyl radical ($OH^{\bullet}$) (this is the most oxidising free radical), superoxide radical ($O_2^{\bullet}$) and nitric oxide ($NO^{\bullet}$).

Free radicals can become stable in a number of ways:
• join together with another free radical;
• remove an electron from a non-radical, leaving a donor with an unpaired electron;
• donate an electron to a non-radical, creating a recipient that is a free radical;
• remove a hydrogen atom from a C–H bond, leaving the C with an unpaired electron (these commonly react with oxygen to form a peroxyl radical, e.g. in lipid peroxidation; see Figure 28.1).

Most of the above initiate a chain reaction, which can be damaging, unless terminated or prevented. Damage can occur to DNA, biological membranes, activation of enzymes and lipoprotein structure

Contributory factors

Iron and copper are potential catalysts for free radical formation and are therefore found in a bound state, generally attached to proteins, to limit their availability. Trauma and inflammatory states cause a reduction in binding, releasing free ions and forming free radicals. However, plasma iron binding capacity increases at this time, to minimise the consequences.

Defence mechanisms

There are many antioxidants present in various compartments that fulfil a protective role. Their distribution is shown in Figure 28.2. In general, an antioxidant is any substance that significantly delays or prevents the oxidation of a target substrate, usually by becoming oxidised itself.

Endogenous antioxidants include a number of enzymes, which require minerals for their action. These include:
• **superoxide dismutase**, which requires *zinc, copper* and *manganese* for activation (depending on location), and neutralises the superoxide radical to hydrogen peroxide and oxygen;
• **glutathione peroxidase**, which is a *selenium-* and *glutathione-*requiring enzyme, and reduces peroxides to water; the glutathione is generated in a reaction requiring *riboflavin* as a cofactor.

Generation of free radicals

Free radicals are generated continuously by several processes:
• Metabolic processes in the electron transport chain, catalysed by metal ions (such as copper and iron).
• Defence mechanisms of the inflammatory process – white cells generate free radicals to kill ingested bacteria in phagocytosis, or secrete free radicals into the surrounding tissues to destroy damaged tissue. Areas of ischaemic or damaged tissue may contain high levels of free radicals.
• Dissociation of oxygen from haemoglobin.
• Exposure to cigarette smoke, sunlight, certain chemicals and high oxygen tension; excess antioxidants may have a pro-oxidant action.

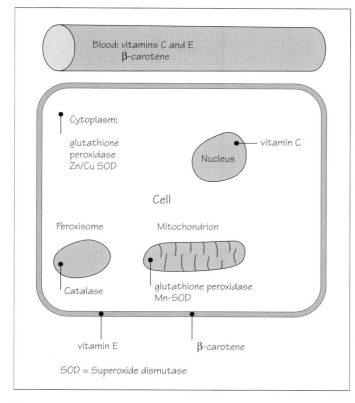

Fig. 28.2 Distribution of antioxidant molecules in cells and blood.

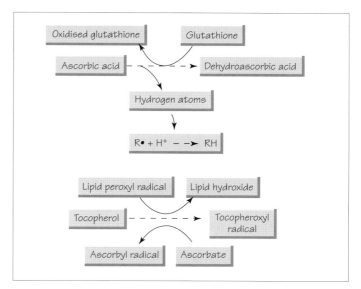

Fig. 28.3 Interactions between glutathione, vitamin C and vitamin E during antioxidant activity.

• **catalase**, which also removes hydrogen peroxide, and is a haem-containing protein, therefore requiring *iron*.

In addition, there are *exogenously* derived antioxidants, of which vitamin C, vitamin E and the carotenoids are the most important.

Vitamin C, a water-soluble vitamin, is important in the *aqueous environment* of the cell and plasma, as an effective scavenger of a wide range of free radicals.

It donates an electron to the free radical, deactivating it, and itself becomes an ascorbyl radical. This is regenerated back to ascorbate, using glutathione, without causing oxidative damage itself.

Particularly high concentrations of vitamin C are found in white blood cells, the eye and in lung tissue, where the protective antioxidant effect is critical against high levels of free radicals, oxygen and pollutants respectively.

Vitamin E is the major antioxidant found in the *lipid environment*; especially in the lipid layers of biological membranes. Particularly

large concentrations occur in organs exposed to highly oxygenated blood, such as the lungs and heart.

• The vitamin (as tocopherol) is able to donate a hydrogen to a lipid peroxyl radical, to produce a lipid hydroperoxide and a tocopheroxyl radical.

• The latter has low reactivity, thus breaking the chain reaction; the tocopheroxyl radical can be regenerated to tocopherol by ubiquinone, vitamin C or glutathione (which also requires glutathione peroxidase, and therefore selenium) (Figure 28.3).

Signs of vitamin E deficiency include neurological and muscular damage, and may be attributable to the effects of free radicals on membranes.

Carotenoids have been shown to quench singlet oxygen by absorbing the excitation energy, and forming a harmless carotenoid, thus removing the potential for free radical formation. The major carotenoid normally considered is β-carotene, which is converted in the body to retinol. There are many other carotenoids with antioxidant properties, including lycopene and lutein.

Dietary vitamin C

Vitamin C is mainly obtained in the diet from plant foods, with rich sources among both fruit (citrus fruits, berries, summer fruits) and vegetables (peppers, broccoli, cauliflower, tomatoes). If potatoes are eaten regularly they can provide a consistent intake.

Cooking losses can be high.

Consuming at least five servings of fruit and vegetables per day (400 g) is an effective way of achieving adequate vitamin C status, especially if some are eaten raw.

Dietary vitamin E

Vitamin E is supplied by vegetable oils, and from whole-grain cereals, which contain the vitamin in the germ of the grain.

Green leafy vegetables, some fruit and nuts also supply vitamin E.

Manufactured foods, such as potato or cereal products, may provide some vitamin E, included as fat in the recipe.

Animal foods are not important sources of vitamin E, although eggs, fish and poultry may contain small amounts.

Carotenoids in the diet

Carotenoids are found in plant foods as red or yellow pigments. Rich sources include carrots, dark-green leafy vegetables, broccoli, red peppers, tomatoes, apricots, peaches and mango.

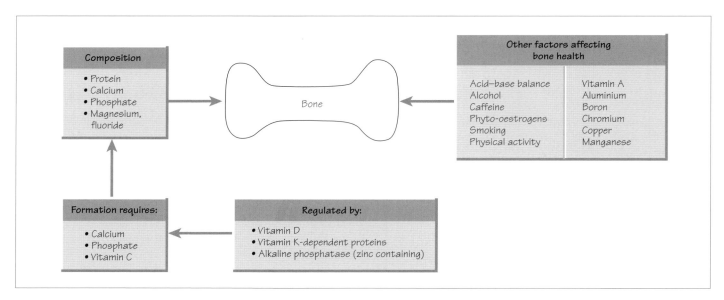

Fig. 29.1 Overview of factors involved in bone formation and bone health.

Aims

(1) To study the factors involved in the formation of bone.
(2) To identify the role of calcium in the formation and maintenance of the skeleton.

The human skeleton

The skeleton serves several key roles:
• provides the framework to which is attached the musculature of the body;
• provides protection for the more delicate organs, such as the brain and organs of the chest;
• acts as a reservoir for some minerals, and is important in acid–base regulation;
• is a site of blood cell synthesis.

Composition of bone

Bone can be classified as cortical (compact) or trabecular (spongy), with corresponding structural and metabolic characteristics (Table 29.1). Bones comprise an extracellular organic matrix made up of proteins (predominantly *collagen*), on which inorganic substances are deposited.
• The **proteins** play important roles in regulating the mineralization of bone, and include alkaline phosphatase, which is **zinc** containing, and gamma-carboxylated proteins, which are dependent on **vitamin K**.
• The major mineral constituents of bone are **calcium** and **phosphate**, combined as hydroxyapatite, laid down around collagen fibres to form a rigid structure.
• Trace elements such as **magnesium**, **fluoride** or **strontium** may occasionally replace calcium in the crystalline structure, changing the size of the crystals and affecting strength and solubility.

Bone formation, resorption and remodelling

• **Bone formation:** is carried out by *osteoblasts*; continues throughout life but takes place predominantly until the late teens, then at a reduced rate up to the age of 25–30.
• **Bone resorption:** is effected by *osteoclasts*; continues throughout life, increasing after the age of 30; accelerates in the 10–15-year period after the menopause in women. In men the gradual rate continues into old age. This loss of bone mass results in osteoporosis. When the loss of bone mass reaches a critical point, the bone may fracture on stress or impact.
• **Osteocytes** are the most numerous cells, embedded throughout the bone; they play a role in regulating bone metabolism, for growth, repair and supplying calcium to plasma.
• Variations in the remodelling process can result in changes to bone density and mass. The process of remodelling is under hormonal control by parathyroid hormone, calcitonin and active vitamin D. Growth hormone, glucocorticoids and oestrogen are also involved.

Nutrient involvement in bone health

See Figure 29.1 for an overview.

Calcium

Calcium is the most prevalent mineral, with approximately 1 kg present in the bones of an adult. Bones act as a source of ionised calcium for nerve and muscle function, as well as blood clotting, and plasma levels are maintained within narrow limits.

Nevertheless, the body's requirement for calcium varies with the rate of bone development, rather than metabolic needs. The daily need

Table 29.1 The main types of bone found in the human body.

Type of bone	Amount and main locations	Main characteristics
Cortical (or compact)	80–85% of total bone; in long bones	Very dense, slowly metabolised
Trabecular (or spongy)	15–20% of total bone; in vertebrae, flat bones and ends of long bones	More readily metabolised and therefore more susceptible to fracture Forms a mesh of calcified trabeculae (a scaffold), blood cells formed within the spaces, which are filled with marrow

Main sources of calcium in Western diets

- Milk and dairy products (tofu set with calcium or calcium-enriched soya milk are alternative sources for vegetarians).
- Cereals and cereal products (may be fortified with calcium).
- Green leafy vegetables.
- Small fish (eaten with their bones).
- Some seeds and nuts are additional sources, but their importance depends on the amounts eaten, as levels are lower than in dairy products.
- Hard water may provide an important source of calcium in some geographical locations.

is at its highest during the peak growth spurt of adolescence, reaching 300 mg/day, and therefore calcium intakes are especially critical at this time, to ensure adequate mineralisation of the bone.

Table 29.2 A summary of factors affecting calcium absorption.

Factors promoting calcium absorption	Factors inhibiting calcium absorption
Vitamin D	Phytate (e.g. in whole-grain cereals, chapattis)
Lactose	Oxalate (e.g. from spinach, beetroot, chocolate)
Dietary protein	Use of antacids
Non-digestible oligosaccharides	Unabsorbed dietary fats
Acidic conditions in jejunum	Excessive intakes of dietary fibre
	Large intakes of phosphoric acid (e.g. in carbonated drinks)

Calcium absorption is influenced by a number of promoting and inhibitory factors (Table 29.2). Unabsorbed calcium, together with that secreted into the digestive tract, is lost in the faeces. It can bind to fats in the digestive tract, forming soaps, and reducing fat absorption. Equally, fat malabsorption can remove calcium from the large intestine.

Calcium balance can be achieved at a variety of levels of calcium intake, demonstrating that calcium absorption is well controlled to match the needs of the body (Table 29.3). Even at low intake levels, calcium balance remains neutral. Only in the adolescent, where needs are increased, is there a positive balance, achieved by increasing efficiency of absorption and reducing urinary loss.

Calcium balance is regulated by activity at:
- the gut (absorption);
- the kidney (excretion);
- the bone (mobilisation and deposition).

These sites are controlled by feedback mechanisms through an interplay of hormones, including the activated form of vitamin D. Serum calcium levels only become abnormal if there is a failure of this homeostatic mechanism, and not as a result of changes in dietary calcium intakes.

Table 29.3 Calcium balance at differing levels of intake.

Calcium intake (mg)	Faecal excretion (mg)	Urinary excretion (mg)
1500	1200	300
1000 (adult)	825	175
1000 (adolescent)	675	125
400	300	100

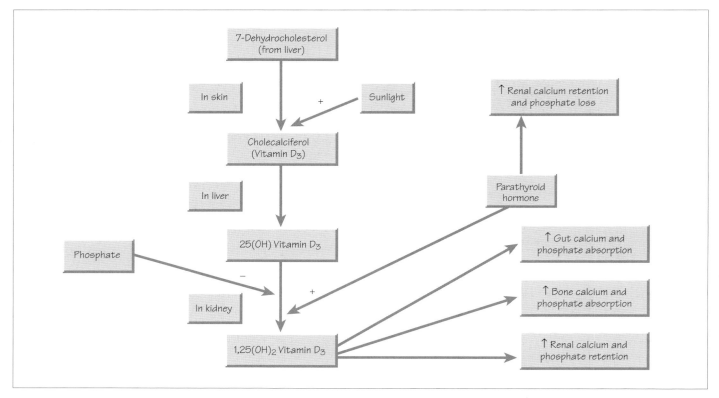

Fig. 30.1 Interaction between vitamin D, calcium and phosphate (reproduced with permission from Gibney (2004) *Public Health Nutrition*, Blackwell Publishing).

Aims

(1) To identify the role of other micronutrients in the formation and maintenance of the skeleton and their interaction with calcium.

Vitamin D

Vitamin D is essential in the regulation of calcium balance, and a deficiency will result in inadequate bone mineralisation, as seen in rickets (in children) and osteomalacia (in adults). Although the amounts of collagen matrix are normal in these deficiency states, the bone is softer, particularly at the growth points, and is susceptible to deformation. This results in the characteristic bow legs or knock knees and deformed spine of rickets seen in children, and back and joint pain in adults, with difficulty in walking.

Metabolic role

The active form of vitamin D is 1,25-dihydroxycalcitriol, which is produced in two stages by the addition of hydroxyl groups.

The first stage occurs in the liver, yielding 25-hydroxycalcitriol, which is the form commonly measured in the blood.

The second stage of activation occurs in the kidney; this is regulated by parathyroid hormone secreted in response to falling plasma calcium levels. Overall, the effect of active vitamin D is to raise plasma calcium levels by:
- increasing absorption of calcium at the gut, via a calcium-binding protein (calbindin-D);
- promoting calcium reabsorption at the kidneys;
- modulating the mobilisation and deposition of calcium and phosphorus in the bones.

A summary of the main interactions between vitamin D and calcium balance is shown in Figure 30.1.

Sources of vitamin D

Vitamin D is supplied in a number of foods in the diet:
- dairy products (levels may be lower in low-fat versions, unless fortified);
- spreading fats;
- oily fish;
- meat and eggs;
- fortified breakfast cereals.

For most people the major source of vitamin D is by synthesis in the skin, from 7-dehydrocholesterol, on exposure to ultraviolet light (290–320 nm wavelength).

In northern latitudes, sunlight of this wavelength reaches the earth only between March and October, so no synthesis occurs during the winter months.

Dietary intake is important in those individuals who do not spend time out of doors, and supplementation may be necessary.

Table 30.1 Possible causes of low vitamin D status.

Mechanism	Reason(s)
Inadequate intake	Few dietary sources; strict vegetarian diet
	Low levels in formula milk or weaning diet
Poor absorption	A fat-soluble vitamin, absorption may be hindered by fat malabsorption conditions, as well as removal of endogenously synthesised vitamin D secreted into the gut
	Excretion increased by alcohol and anticonvulsant drugs
Low levels of skin synthesis	Little skin exposure: housebound, skin covered, use of sun creams
	Dark skin pigmentation, reduced synthesis with ageing
Poor activation of the vitamin	Liver disease or kidney disease
	Parathyroid disease

Deficiency of vitamin D may arise for a number of reasons (Table 30.1).

Phosphorus

Phosphorus is present as phosphate, and is the second major mineral in bone. In addition, phosphate is widely distributed throughout the tissues in biologically vital compounds such as ATP and nucleic acids.

Regulation of plasma phosphate is mainly by renal excretion, which balances with dietary intake and is also influenced by parathyroid hormone and therefore calcium levels. The two minerals are closely associated to maintain a constant ratio.

Depletion of serum phosphate can result in poor mineralisation, but this is most likely to happen in disease states or starvation.

Other minerals and vitamins

Magnesium

Magnesium is involved in the formation of bone crystals and in parathyroid hormone function, but there is little evidence that changes within normal limits in magnesium intake have a major effect on bone health.

Vitamin A

Large intakes of vitamin A have been associated with changes to the bones, including thickening of the long bones and hypercalcaemia, associated with increased bone resorption. It is currently unclear if vitamin A has a role in normal skeletal health.

Diet and phosphates

Phosphates are widely distributed in the diet in both animal and plant foods, and are also used as an additive by the food industry.

There is some concern about high phosphate intakes from carbonated drinks, and their potential to impair calcium absorption from the gut, with a consequent effect on bone mineralisation. However, evidence is equivocal.

Excessive intakes of vitamin A, taken as supplements, have been reported to cause bone demineralisation.

Vitamin C

Vitamin C is needed for formation of the hydroxylated amino acids lysine and proline, which are essential for the cross-linking in collagen. Bone fractures occur in scurvy, but it is possible that even at subclinical levels of vitamin C deficiency, there is an increased risk. This has been reported in smokers.

Vitamin K

This is needed for the gamma-carboxylation of glutamate residues to form three key proteins found in bone, including osteocalcin, which has high calcium-binding activity. Inverse relationships have been identified in older people between vitamin K status and fracture risk.

Potassium

Potassium has been proposed as an important factor in bone health, and linked to a higher bone mineral density and thus a lower fracture risk. Fruit and vegetables provide a major source of potassium in the diet, and it has been postulated that the *alkaline residues* from fruit and vegetables minimise the demand for buffering salts to be drawn from the bones, avoiding a potential demineralising effect. This is in contrast to the situation where *acid residues*, for example from proteins and cereals, require buffering by ions such as citrate and carbonate from bones.

Other factors

A number of other minerals have been proposed as playing an important part in bone metabolism. These include zinc, copper, boron, aluminium, manganese and chromium. More research is needed to clarify their exact role.

In addition other dietary factors are believed to affect bone health. These include:
- alcohol – generally has a negative effect on bone density, via a toxic effect on the osteoblasts;
- caffeine – increases calcium loss in the urine; however, additional milk taken with coffee may offset this effect;
- phyto-oestrogens – found in soya; have been reported to have a beneficial effect, via a weak oestrogenic action. The amount to be consumed is higher than habitual levels in Western countries.

Lifestyle factors affecting bone, include smoking (which has a negative effect on bone density), and physical activity, which is beneficial and stimulates bone formation and mineralisation at the sites of mechanical strain. Conversely, immobilisation and lack of activity cause a reduction in bone mass.

Concerns about the increasing prevalence of osteoporosis have focused attention on the role of nutritional and non-nutritional factors in bone health. Attention to diet, within healthy eating guidelines, can provide the nutrients necessary for formation and maintenance of bone.

31 Alcohol in the diet

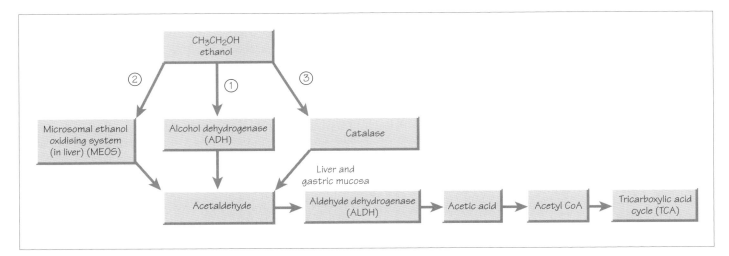

Fig. 31.1 Metabolism of alcohol.

Aims

(1) To consider sources of alcohol and quantities consumed.
(2) To study metabolism of alcohol and consequences of excessive consumption.

Alcohol is not essential in the diet although almost 90% of the UK population consume it at some time. The main clinical risk factor associated with heavy drinking is cirrhosis of the liver. Rates are increasingly rapidly in the UK.

Alcohol consumption affects every system in the body, especially the gastrointestinal, cardiovascular and nervous systems.

There are social consequences of excessive alcohol intake, including violence, accidents, suicide and family breakdown. Absence from work results in economic consequences.

Measurement of alcohol consumption

A 'unit' of alcohol is defined in the UK as 8 g or 10 mL of ethanol (in the USA it is 12 g of alcohol).

Guidelines on the numbers of units in *standard alcoholic drinks* were issued some years ago by the UK's Health Education Authority (HEA). Drinks now available are more diverse and stronger, leading to confusion about numbers of units (Table 31.1).

Table 31.1 Numbers of units in commonly available drinks.

Alcoholic drink	Quantity	Strength (% alcohol)	Units
Standard strength beer[a]	½ pint (284 mL)	3.5	1
Premium beer	½ pint (284 mL)	5	1.5
Strong beer	½ pint (284 mL)	6.5	2
Export strength (cans)	440 mL	8.6	3.75
Single 'shot' of spirits[a]	25 mL	40	1
Double 'shot'	50 mL	40	2
Glass of wine[a]	125 mL	8	1
Small 'bar' glass of wine	175 mL	11	2
Large 'bar' glass of full-bodied wine	250 mL	13	3
Alcopop (bottle)	275 mL	5	1.4

[a]Drinks used in setting original advice on alcohol units.

Government recommendations for safe alcohol intake are no more than 3–4 units per day for men and 2–3 units for women (binge drink-

Social factors

Alcohol consumption varies across the UK population, so that:
- men drink twice as much as women overall (differences in younger age groups are less than this);
- single men drink more than married men;
- consumption is highest in the young adult age group, in the form of teenage binge drinking;
- in general, less affluent people drink more than the better-off, although the latter drink more regularly;
- consumption declines with age.

Liver metabolism of alcohol

Within the liver, three main metabolic pathways have been demonstrated (Figure 31.1); all produce acetaldehyde.
- The dominant pathway (1) involves the zinc-containing enzyme alcohol dehydrogenase (ADH), found in liver cytoplasm. This is the main rate-limiting step. The accumulation of acetaldehyde leads to headaches and cutaneous flushing.
- The microsomal ethanol-oxidising system (MEOS) (2) normally metabolises up to 20% of ingested alcohol; it becomes more active in chronic alcoholics. Alcohol stimulates the development of microsomal membranes, where cytochrome P450 (a vitamin C requiring factor) is induced.
- A third (relatively insignificant) pathway involves the enzyme catalase found in many cells of the body (3).

ing is defined as consuming twice this daily amount in one day) per day. In a week, intakes should not exceed 21 units for men and 14 units for women, and there should be alcohol-free days.

Weekly alcohol intakes exceeding 55 units for men and 35 units for women are regarded as being 'likely to do harm'.

Metabolism of alcohol

The rate at which alcohol is metabolised varies considerably and is related to body size. In a healthy young male it may be 8–10 g (i.e. 1 unit) per hour.

Women experience greater rises in blood alcohol levels because they have a greater fat content, less body water and generally lower body weight, leading to a higher concentration of alcohol.

Metabolism is also affected by:
* genetic factors;
* lean body mass;
* other foods in the diet;
* previous history of alcohol intake (rate is higher in chronic alcoholics).

Alcohol and energy balance

Alcohol yields 29 kJ (7 kcal) per gram. If drunk in addition to a normal food intake, the extra energy is likely to cause weight gain.

This is not always the case; alcohol metabolised via the MEOS system produces little ATP; rather the process of oxidation leads to heat production, which is dissipated and not stored.

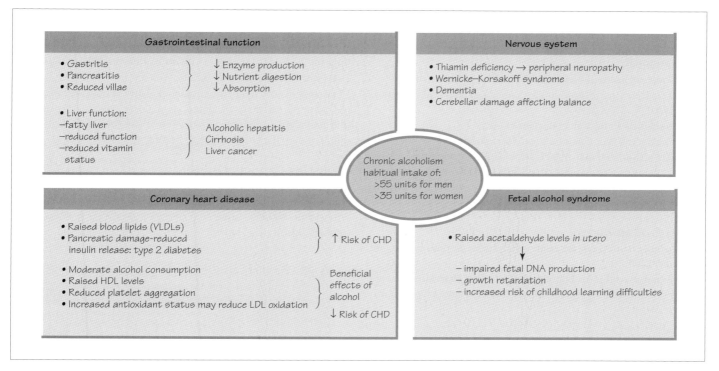

Fig. 31.2 Health aspects of alcohol consumption.

Nutritional consequences of alcohol abuse

* **Fat metabolism** in the liver becomes abnormal. The large amounts of NADH and NADPH produced by metabolism stimulate fat synthesis, which leads to high levels of circulating VLDL. In heavy drinkers the liver increases in size due to the accumulation of excess fat, eventually leading to chronic inflammation.
* Control of **blood glucose** levels is less effective. This reflects reduced insulin production and reduced gluconeogenesis. Hypoglycaemic episodes, resulting in 'blackouts', may occur.
* Although protein catabolism is unaffected, **protein synthesis** is reduced. Tissue repair is compromised and digestive enzyme production is reduced.
* Activation of B vitamins is compromised by liver disease.
  –Low status of **niacin**, **riboflavin** and **pyridoxine** may lead to diarrhoea, dermatitis and psychological problems.

–Reduced folate absorption leads to megaloblastic anaemia
–Reduced thiamin absorption, associated with vomiting and diarrhoea, and increased demand for thiamin results in deficiency, with peripheral neuropathy. In its severe form, psychological disturbance, loss of memory and psychosis (Wernicke–Korsakoff syndrome) may develop.
* Production of **vitamin K** cofactors in the liver ceases, affecting blood clotting.
* Alcohol induces the breakdown of active forms of **vitamin D**.
* **Zinc** is a cofactor for alcohol dehydrogenase. Levels may be reduced, which will compromise alcohol metabolism, decrease wound healing, dull the sense of taste and reduce immune function.
* **Iron** status may vary; spirits provide no iron but some wines and beers do contain iron. Blood loss due to intestinal mucosal irritation may lead to iron depletion.

32 Fluids in the diet

Aims

(1) To consider the need for water in the body and the role of fluid.
(2) To explore the ways in which fluids can contribute to fluid balance and to nutrition.

Water makes up 50–60% of total body weight of an average adult, and even small reductions in levels of hydration have serious consequences for normal functions. Water content is higher in males than females due to a higher percentage of lean mass, which contains more water than does fat. Humans cannot survive beyond about ten days without water.

Water is required for the following processes:
- ingestion, digestion and absorption of food including the production of various secretions, movement along the digestive tract and elimination of waste;
- transport of nutrients and metabolites in solution; metabolic processes occurring in fluid environments; establishing osmotic gradients;
- maintenance of moist mucous membranes;
- maintenance of blood volumes and haematocrit, extracellular and intracellular fluid volumes, which affect tissue osmolarity;
- renal function, which is dependent on adequate perfusion pressure;
- body temperature regulation by sweat loss.

Fluid balance

Fluid balance represents the relationship between fluid intake and fluid loss (Table 32.1).

Fluid intake is largely under the control of the individual; people relying on others for fluid may be unable to determine their intake.

Fluid is lost from the body in a number of ways, which are normally outside individual control.

Maintenance of normal hydration

No recommended intake for daily fluid is recorded in tables of dietary reference values (DRVs); most sedentary adults in a temperate climate need about 1200–1500 mL/day. This assumes a further 1000 mL of fluid is being obtained from food, resulting in a total fluid gain of 35 mL/kg body weight per day. Consequences of dehydration are summarised in Table 32.2.

Dehydration

The thirst mechanism is triggered by a fall in body fluid volume normally associated with a rise in osmolality. These signals to consume additional fluid appear after the onset of dehydration. Thus anticipatory fluid consumption may be the only way to prevent dehydration, and fluid consumption should become a habit. Although the prevalence of mild dehydration is not known, a significant proportion of the population may be affected (Table 32.3).

Water loss from the body

Urine

Daily urine production (diuresis) closely follows levels of hydration. Pale, straw-coloured urine indicates good hydration; small volumes of dark-yellow urine indicate significant levels of dehydration.

Dietary factors that influence diuresis

- High-sodium and -protein diets increase the solute load and therefore obligatory urine loss and require compensatory increases in fluid intake.
- Caffeine is a methylxanthine (found in coffee, tea and colas and some high-energy drinks) and is chemically related to theobromine and theophylline found in tea and chocolate. These have a diuretic action; however, at doses of <300 mg/day the level of diuresis is offset by the volume of fluid ingested. In practice this means that caffeine consumption will not lead to a significant level of dehydration.
- Alcohol produces a diuresis. Consuming neat spirit could lead to negative fluid balance, but alcohol in beer will result in a positive balance because of the fluid accompanying the alcohol in the drink.

Table 32.1 A summary of average values for fluid gain and loss per day for a healthy individual leading a sedentary life (note values vary depending on circumstances).

Water gain – route	Water gain – volume (mL)	Water loss – route	Water loss – volume (mL)
Water in food	1000	Urine	1300
Metabolic water	350	Faeces	100
Drinks	1200	Skin	750
		Lungs	400
Totals	2550		2550

Table 32.2 Summary of consequences of dehydration.

Degree of dehydration	Amount of fluid deficit	Consequences	Comments
Mild	500–1000 mL; 1–2% body weight	May affect cognitive function	May reduce accuracy in performance
Mild to moderate	1000–3500 mL; 2–5% body weight	Headaches, cognitive impairment, nausea	Substantial detrimental effect on performance in sporting activity; affects temperature regulation
Severe	>6% body weight	Pyrexia, tachycardia, dizziness, weakness	Loss of physical performance skill
Life threatening	10%	Raised blood pressure, renal failure, coma and death	

Table 32.3 Population groups at risk of dehydration.

Group at possible risk	Reason(s) for vulnerability
Young children	Poorly developed thirst mechanism/lack of awareness Dependence on others for fluid supply Relatively low body water volume Large surface area for water evaporation
Dependent elderly people	Possible confusion about fluid intake Dependence on others for fluid supply Relatively low body water volume Possible drug therapy (e.g. diuretics) Poor food intake, little metabolic water produced Reluctance to drink because of limited mobility to use lavatory
Subjects with raised body temperature	Increased losses through skin (sweating) and lungs (rapid breathing) Poor appetite, little food intake Possible losses from GI tract in vomiting/diarrhoea Poor thirst mechanism/provision of fluids
Sportspeople	Large sweat losses to maintain body temperature Increased respiration and lung losses Inability/unwillingness to consume fluid during exercise
People working in heat	Large sweat losses

Faeces

Fluid loss in the faeces is small (about 100 mL/day); this can rise to 2000 mL/day in diarrhoeal diseases and represents a major threat to life. Abuse of laxatives can result in large losses, and lead to dehydration.

Skin

Water loss through skin occurs continuously. Children are particularly at risk because their surface:volume ratio is considerably higher than adults. Normal levels of water loss can be doubled in heat, where sweating occurs for heat regulation (it is estimated that sweat loss increases by 500 mL/day for each 1°C rise in body temperature). Even moderate exercise increases sweat losses to 1000–3000 mL/h.

Lungs

For effective gas exchange in the lungs, inhaled air must be moistened, and exhaled air therefore contains water vapour. Dry climates, air-conditioned offices and high-altitude situations also encourage this form of water loss.

Water gain by the body

Metabolism and water in food

Small amounts of water are produced during metabolic processes. Water is also ingested with food:

- some foods are semi-liquid (e.g. yogurts, soups and ice cream);
- many foods contain a high percentage of water (e.g. fruit and vegetables);
- 'dry' foods such as cereals, bread, dairy products and meat contain some water.

Drinks

Consumption of water from drinks is very variable. The choice of drink may make an important contribution to nutrient intake (Table 32.4).

Table 32.4 Possible nutritional contribution from drinks.

Type of drink	Possible nutrient contribution	Comments
Water	Calcium from hard water; fluoride in some areas Bottled water may provide a range of minerals	Provision of water in schools and workplaces encourages consumption
Soft drinks, including carbonated and dilutables (squash/cordial)	May contain high levels of sugar; cola drinks contain phosphoric acid	Can lead to passive overconsumption of energy. Damage to teeth and bones from phosphates
Fruit juices	Provide vitamin C and some phytochemicals	Sugar content and acidity detrimental to teeth if not diluted
Tea and coffee	Antioxidants and fluoride in tea, especially green tea Milk contributes to nutrients	Often consumed regularly throughout the day, useful sources of hydration
Milk	Provides vitamins (A, B_{12} and riboflavin) and minerals (calcium, iodine, phosphorus, magnesium, potassium and zinc)	Flavoured milks, milk shakes and probiotics are increasingly popular; some contain added sugar
Alcohol	Beers may contain some B vitamins; wines are a source of antioxidants	Further information on alcohol is in Chapter 31

33 Nutrition and the gastrointestinal tract I

Aims

(1) To review the general functions of the gastrointestinal tract (GI) tract.

(2) To consider some disorders of the GI tract that impact on nutritional status.

(3) To consider the interdependence of the upper GI tract and nutritional status.

Food enters the body via the mouth at the start of the GI tract; throughout its length an enormous variety and complexity of products are converted into simple nutrients. From here, the nutrients are absorbed into the body across a very large surface area composed of villi and microvilli.

In order to perform its role adequately, the GI tract itself must be supplied with energy and nutrients. Nutritional deficiencies that affect cell division will have a rapid impact on the GI tract, as the cells here have a short life span and undergo continuous replication. Thus deficiencies of folate, vitamin B_{12}, riboflavin and niacin will all affect the efficiency of digestion and absorption.

General functions

The GI tract fulfils a number of roles, only some of which are directly involved with the digestion of food. These are summarised in Table 33.1.

Because of the diversity of roles of the GI tract, a number of disorders have a potential impact on the overall function. These are summarised in Table 33.2.

Interrelationship between nutrition and function of the regions of the upper GI tract

The mouth

Ingestion of food is crucial for normal nutrition. The teeth and jaws initiate the breakdown process by the action of chewing, whereas the secretion of saliva contributes to the sense of taste, lubricates the food for swallowing and provides some digestive enzymes.

- **Teeth** are important for chewing, and although edentulous subjects can grind food with their gums, studies of older adults without their

Table 33.1 A summary of the roles of the GI tract and consequences if these are compromised.

Role of GI tract	Specific functions	Impact on overall health if role is compromised
Processing of food	Ingestion, chewing, swallowing Digestion, absorption Excretion of waste material	Nutritional deficiencies, which are likely to affect the function of the GI tract as well as other parts of the body
Regulation of feeding behaviour	Signals arise from mouth, stomach and small intestine; include chemical and neural signals	Overall food intake may be poorly controlled if signals absent
Protective and barrier function	Low stomach pH is bactericidal Mucus coating Innate immune system secretions, include: lysozyme, antibacterial enzymes, mast cells and macrophages Adaptive immunodefences, include production of immunoglobulins and antibodies Secretion of cytokines and interleukins	Produces a balance of responses, to neutralise harmful organisms, but maintain beneficial flora Inappropriate antibody responses to foods must be avoided If these fail, hypersensitivity may develop, with chronic GI conditions

Table 33.2 Disorders of the GI tract that may affect digestion and absorption.

Disorder	Aetiology	Symptoms/treatment
Coeliac disease	Sensitivity to gluten in cereals; may be diagnosed in infancy or not appear until later in life	Atrophy of villi of the small intestine, resulting in malabsorption and potential malnutrition if not treated. Improved by following a gluten-free diet
Crohn's disease (CD)	Inflammatory condition affecting terminal ileum and colon, but with normal areas between sites. Some genetic links but triggered by environmental factors, increased by smoking	Diarrhoea or constipation. Low-grade chronic fever. May be associated with anaemia, B_{12} deficiency Treated with anti-inflammatory or immunosuppressive drugs May have some success with probiotics
Ulcerative colitis	Similar to CD but confined to colon, and continuous. Does not extend through bowel wall	Diarrhoea; other symptoms similar to CD. Risk of development of colon cancer Treatment as for CD
Irritable bowel syndrome (IBS)	No obvious pathology, may exhibit increased motility, sensitivity to specific foods, altered bowel flora	Pain or discomfort relating to GI tract, bloating, but with no obvious pathology Treatment varies with individual and may include behavioural therapy, food elimination, and probiotics. Increased fibre intake is of benefit in some cases

own teeth show that nutritional intakes are poorer.

• Nutrients of importance for healthy teeth include: **calcium**, **phosphorus** and **protein**; **fluoride** increases strength and resistance to decay. Fermentable **carbohydrate** intake, in forms that adhere to the teeth, and consumed between meals is a major contributory factor to decay, and ultimately loss of teeth.

• The **sense of taste** allows food to be recognised, and decisions made about its palatability and consumption. Gastric secretions begin as a result of reflexes triggered by eating. Taste sensitivity is affected by nutrient deficiencies, most notably **vitamin A** and **zinc**; some drugs also affect taste and therefore possibly food consumption.

• **Saliva flow** can diminish with ageing as well as with drug treatment and disease, and artificial saliva may be used to help chewing and swallowing in these situations.

The stomach

Food is liquidised in the stomach by pressure and a churning action, and released at a controlled rate into the duodenum. This rate is determined by feedback mechanisms from the intestines that monitor the composition of stomach contents; the most important of these is cholecystokinin (CCK).

Key features of the secretions in the stomach are: hydrochloric acid, proteolytic enzymes, intrinsic factor and mucus. The presence of food rapidly elevates the pH to approximately 4.5. Gastric acidity serves to:

• provide the correct environment for the activation of proteolytic enzymes and start the process of protein digestion;

• solubilise the divalent minerals in the diet (especially calcium and iron);

• prevent the conversion of nitrates into nitrites, which form carcinogenic nitrosamines;

• release vitamin B_{12} from its protein binding, for attachment to intrinsic factor and later absorption.

Reduced gastric acidity will therefore interfere with absorption of some minerals and of vitamin B_{12}. For example, use of antacid indigestion remedies will raise the pH and therefore limit the solubilisation of minerals.

Excessive **alcohol intake** also damages the gastric mucosa, resulting in chronic gastritis, and affecting normal digestive processes and therefore nutritional status.

Nutrition and the gastrointestinal tract II

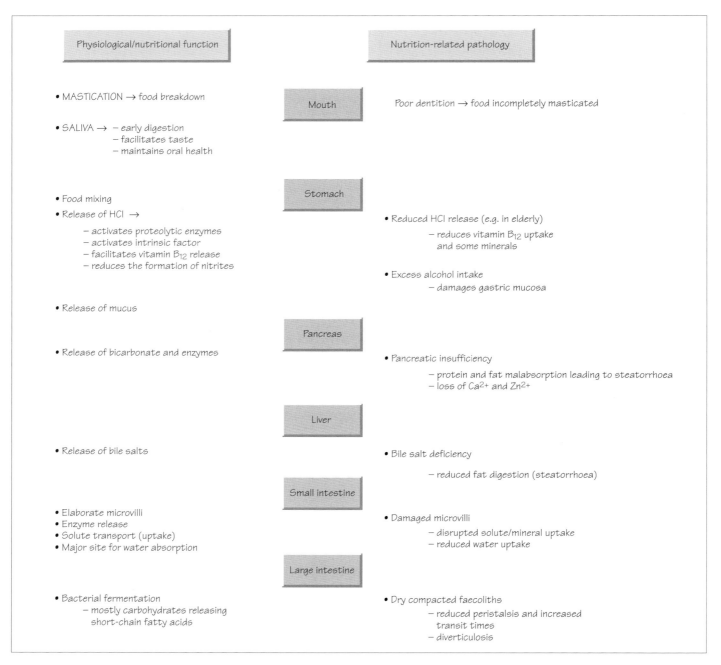

Fig. 34.1 Summary of the physiological/nutritional aspects of gastrointestinal function and nutrition-related pathology.

Aims

(1) To consider the interdependence of the lower GI tract and nutritional status.

The small intestine

This is the major site of digestion, brought about by bicarbonate and enzyme secretions from the pancreas, and enzymes located in the brush borders of the microvilli.

In addition, bile manufactured by the liver and released from the gall bladder enters the small intestine at this point.

Bile acids are required for the emulsification of lipids prior to fat digestion, so failure of bile production or secretion will also compromise fat digestion and result in steatorrhoea. This may be the result of liver disease, or blockage of the bile ducts preventing release of bile.

Pancreatic insufficiency

All three macronutrients are digested by pancreatic enzymes. Pancreatic insufficiency therefore will have a profound effect on nutritional status. This is likely to include:

- generalised macronutrient undernutrition, predominantly relating to **protein and fat malabsorption**;
- **fat-soluble vitamin malabsorption**;
- steatorrhoea, also causing **loss of calcium** from the body due to its binding to fatty acids;
- **zinc deficiency** due to absence of zinc-binding protein to facilitate absorption.

In cystic fibrosis, where pancreatic secretions are blocked by mucus, ingestion of enzymes to digest food is necessary to prevent nutritional deficiency. Nevertheless macronutrient intakes larger than normal are required to compensate for the reduced digestion.

Absorption

This is a key function of the small intestine; under normal circumstances there is a mixture of passive and active transport systems in operation for the absorption of the products of macronutrient digestion (see Table 34.1 for summary).

The surface area of the small intestine is very large, derived from the villi and microvilli on its surface, to facilitate the absorption process. Damage or flattening of these has serious consequences for absorption. The main example of a condition where this occurs is **coeliac disease**; other malabsorption states may also be associated with flattened villi.

Water absorption

This is critical in the small intestine: daily some 8 litres is reabsorbed here, deriving from digestive secretions as well as food intake. Only approximately 100 mL/h enters the large intestine.

Water follows solute absorption, principally glucose and sodium, but gene studies suggest there may also be specific water transporters involved. If solutes are not absorbed, water remains in the intestine and moves through to the large intestine, where it will result in osmotic diarrhoea.

Malabsorption of sugars, for example lactose, artificial sweeteners such as xylitol, and lactulose (a synthetic disaccharide used as a laxative), can all have this effect.

The large intestine

Undigested or unabsorbed food residues and endogenous substances reach the large intestine, together with approximately 1–1.5 L of water. Water absorption occurs with solutes such as short-chain fatty acids and active transport of sodium. Some water absorption may be under hormonal control.

Any breakdown of residues in the colon occurs largely by the action of bacteria found here. This includes:

- proteins, which are broken down to volatile amines;
- carbohydrates, mainly broken down to short-chain fatty acids (acetic, propionic and butyric), carbon dioxide, hydrogen and methane;
- long-chain fatty acids are generally not fermented, and therefore result in steatorrhoea;
- phytochemicals and hormone residues may also be broken down here, together with bile acids that escaped absorption in the ileum.

Butyric acid is an important nutrient for the colonocytes, so its synthesis is critical for the health of the colon.

The recognition that the large intestine contains a bacterial flora that may have beneficial effects has led to the study of possible supplementation with bacteria, in the form of probiotics. These are intended to rebalance the bacteria to a more beneficial profile, and eliminate the less desirable strains such as *Escherichia coli* and *Clostridium difficile*. However, results to date have not shown consistent improvements, or lasting effects once treatment is terminated.

The physiological and nutritional relationships along the GI tract are summarised in Figure 34.1.

Colonic bacteria and micronutrients

There is still uncertainty about the nutritional significance of any synthesis of vitamins by the colonic bacteria and their availability to the body:

- vitamin K synthesised here may be of some significance to the body;
- B vitamin synthesis may only be of use to the colonocytes themselves, and not be available to the whole body.

Minerals that had been trapped in dietary fibre matrices may be released here, but it is uncertain whether they are absorbed for whole body use.

Table 34.1 Summary of the absorption of nutrients from the small intestine, and some reasons for failure.

Nutrients	Mechanism of absorption	Possible reasons for failure
Fat-soluble vitamins	Absorbed with fat digestion products; require fat in the diet and normal fat digestion	Pancreatic or biliary insufficiency
Water-soluble vitamins	Generally absorbed by sodium-dependent active transport mechanisms	May become saturated by high intake
Folate	Must be split from conjugates by a zinc-dependent enzyme, then reduced and methylated prior to absorption	Excess amounts of alcohol interfere with the conjugase enzyme activity and therefore reduce folate absorption
Iron and zinc	Require carrier for absorption. Enterocyte binds the transported mineral to a protein, from which it is released into the circulation only as required for metabolism. Unabsorbed mineral is lost when cells sloughed off at end of life cycle	Rapid movement of intestinal contents. Mineral not solubilised. Competition for carrier
Calcium	Carrier activated by vitamin D	Inadequate vitamin D status
Endogenous secretions	Many nutrients secreted as part of digestive process, recycled by absorption with ingested GI contents	

35 Nutrition and the brain I

Aims

(1) To consider the nutritional requirements for the development of the brain.

(2) To describe the nutrients needed for brain function.

A number of aspects of the relationship between the brain and nutrition are considered:

• Adequate nutrition is required by the brain for its development, maintenance and function.

• The brain is also essential for the control of food intake and as such determines the nutritional status of the whole body (see Chapter 36).

• Behaviour may be related to the supply of nutrients to the brain (see Chapter 36).

Much of the discussion about the brain also applies to the spinal cord (together these form the central nervous system, CNS); in addition the peripheral nervous system may also be affected by some of the nutritional factors discussed.

Growth of the brain

The most rapid period of brain growth occurs from mid-gestation to 18 months after birth. At birth the brain accounts for 10% of the body weight; an adult brain weighs about 1.4 kg, and comprises 2% of body weight.

Different components of the brain grow at different rates and have 'critical periods' when growth is most rapid and vulnerable to adverse influence.

Nutritional links in brain development

Although brain *development* may be protected to some extent in fetal life by diversion of nutrients to the brain, there may be long-term consequences for brain *function* (Table 35.1).

One of the most significant changes in composition after birth is a reduction in water content and increase in lipid content, emphasising the importance of lipids.

Nutritional requirements of the brain

Energy – supply of glucose

The energy needs of the brain are normally met by glucose, which is transported into the brain across the blood–brain barrier by a glucose transporter, which is not responsive to insulin. This transport system has a capacity some ten times greater than the actual daily transport of glucose. Active uptake of glucose by the neurons of the brain is matched to their needs by alterations in blood flow.

Food intake and the brain

• *Glucose transport* into the brain is not affected by intake of carbohydrate or energy supply.

• *Hypoglycaemic episodes* can occur when a large dose of insulin is given, or an intake of readily absorbed carbohydrate (e.g. carbonated drink with a high GI), triggers an insulin reaction, reducing glucose levels too much. This may also happen when alcoholic drinks are consumed on an empty stomach. This can result in confusion, coma and death.

• Overnight fasting, not followed by a balanced breakfast meal, may also result in low blood glucose levels. This has led to the belief that *eating breakfast* is important to maintain levels of concentration during the morning. It is particularly promoted for children, whose attention span in school is likely to be affected.

• *Alcohol ingestion* reduces glucose transport into the brain, which probably contributes to the depressant effect of alcohol on the CNS.

• During *starvation,* the brain adapts to the use of ketone bodies derived from fat breakdown for energy, by inducing a ketone body transporter across the blood–brain barrier.

• Blood ketone levels can also be elevated by very high-fat diets, and such *ketogenic diets* have been used successfully by some therapists to treat seizures, as they are believed to reduce neuronal excitability, especially in children. However, adherence to the diet is difficult.

Table 35.1 Summary of the potential associations between early nutrient intake, brain development and possible long-term consequences for brain function.

Nutrient	Role/effect of excess/deficiency
Generalised undernutrition	A smaller brain with a reduced amount of DNA Potential to recover some of the deficit with good nutrition, possibly up to 18 months Neuronal networks may not be as extensive, affecting long-term cognitive performance and behaviour
Lipids	Approximately half of the lipids are present in myelin; adult amounts are present by the age of 4 years Long-chain PUFAs are required for development; breast-fed infants receive higher levels in milk. Some formula milk is fortified with these fatty acids
Copper	Needed for synthesis of myelin
Folate	Low levels can result in neural tube defects, including anencephaly
Iodine	Deficiency results in cretinism and serious learning disabilities
Iron	Severe iron deficiency in infancy results in long-term reductions in cognitive performance
Vitamin A	Excess intakes are teratogenic to brain
Alcohol	Excess intake can result in fetal alcohol syndrome, with developmental changes to organs including the brain, and behavioural and cognitive abnormalities

Table 35.2 Transport of amino acids across the blood–brain barrier.

Main direction of transport	Examples of amino acids carried	Function in brain
From blood into brain	Tryptophan Phenylalanine Methionine Tyrosine Histidine Arginine Lysine (mainly essential amino acids)	Tryptophan used to synthesise serotonin Phenylalanine and tyrosine used for catecholamines Histidine used for histamine synthesis Arginine used in the production of nitric oxide
From brain to blood	Glutamate Aspartate Alanine Glycine Cysteine (mainly nonessential amino acids)	Glutamate is a major neurotransmitter; mainly transported out of brain to prevent excessive excitatory effects Other amino acids may also have excitatory transmitter or cotransmitter roles, and the brain requires a mechanism to prevent excessively high levels being reached

Up to 20% of the body's oxygen requirement is used by the brain.

Protein

The brain requires protein for its own structure, but protein synthesis in the brain does not appear to be related to dietary protein intakes, other than in very early life. However, levels of amino acids in the blood determine their uptake by the various transporters that carry these across the blood–brain barrier (Table 35.2).

Fatty acids

These are required for the synthesis of neuronal cell membranes (Table 35.3).

Vitamins

Water-soluble vitamins are needed to serve as cofactors for a number of key reactions (Table 35.4).

Minerals

Minerals are involved in cofactor roles, in electrical conduction and ionic channels (Table 35.5).

Table 35.3 Role of fatty acids in brain structure and function.

Fatty acid	Role in brain	Specific function
Linoleic acid and α-linolenic acid	Included in membranes as part of phospholipid molecules, which also contain choline	Influence the fluidity of the membrane and functions of associated molecules, such as transporters and receptors
Docosahexaenoic and arachidonic acids	Used in production of prostaglandins and leukotrienes	Regulate second messenger molecules
Balance of n-3 and n-6 acids		May be associated with mental health

Table 35.5 Role of minerals in brain function.

Mineral	Role within the CNS/ peripheral nervous system	Consequences of deficiency/ protective role
Iron	Iron-dependent enzymes needed for neurotransmitter synthesis; possible role in myelination	Effects on cognition and behaviour High levels may contribute to oxidative damage
Copper	Needed as cofactor, e.g. for dopamine β-hydroxylase, used to synthesise noradrenaline	Neurodegeneration seen in Menkes' disease, a rare genetic disorder with very low copper levels. High levels may contribute to oxidative damage

Table 35.4 Role of vitamins in the brain.

Vitamin	Role within the CNS/peripheral nervous system	Consequences of deficiency/protective role
Thiamin	Metabolism of glucose	Deficiency – Wernicke's encephalopathy, with loss of vestibular function, poor nerve conduction, mental confusion. May lead to Korsakoff's syndrome with loss of short-term memory, and degeneration of midbrain, thalamus and cerebellum Peripheral neuropathy affecting nerve fibres
Riboflavin	Oxidation-reduction reactions	Needed for monoamine oxidase synthesis, no evidence of neurotransmitter abnormalities in deficiency
Niacin	Oxidation-reduction reactions	Pellagra associated with depression and dementia, but mechanisms of this unclear
Pyridoxine	Role as cofactor in many amino acid transformations	Role in synthesis of many neurotransmitters; deficiency may lead to depressed mood and, rarely, seizures
Folate	Involved in DNA synthesis, key role in development	Developmentally, linked to neural tube defects. Also associated with depression in adults, mechanism unclear
Vitamin B_{12}	Methylation reaction within nervous system for myelin synthesis	Demyelination of nerve axons and ultimate degeneration. May also protect axons from damage due to toxins
Vitamin C	Cofactor for dopamine β-hydroxylase for noradrenaline synthesis; antioxidant	May be associated with depression; suggested to protect blood vessels in brain from free radical damage and maintain cognitive function
Vitamins B_6, B_{12}, folate	Required for metabolism of homocysteine	High plasma levels of homocysteine may be associated with development of dementia
Vitamin A	Essential role in retina	Night blindness
Vitamin E	Antioxidant role	Protects fatty acids in neuronal membranes; deficiency may be associated with peripheral nerve degeneration; suggested role in protection against Parkinson's disease and Alzheimer's disease

36 Nutrition and the brain II

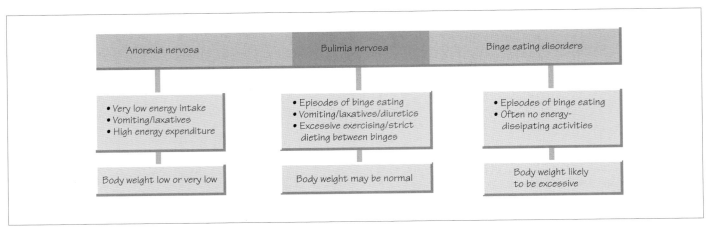

Fig. 36.1 Spectrum of eating disorders resulting in weight changes.

Aims

(1) To consider the role of the brain in control of food intake.
(2) To review the potential role of nutrition in behavioural aspects of brain function.
(3) To consider eating disorders.

Role of the brain in control of food intake

The hypothalamus plays an integrative role in the control of food intake (see Chapter 21). Elements that are involved include the following:

• Information originating from the mouth and senses, the stomach and intestines is conveyed to the hypothalamus via both nervous and chemical signals.
• Numerous gut peptides play key roles in regulation of hunger and feeding; some of these are also found in the brain.
• Metabolic activity in the liver and end products released from it into the circulation, contribute further to regulation.
• One of the key signals is via leptin, a hormone produced predominantly from adipose tissue that acts on the hypothalamus to induce satiety.
• In addition, neurotransmitters acting within the brain are thought to regulate preferences for particular macronutrients. Serotonin may influence the balance between carbohydrate and protein intakes. Noradrenaline and opiates are also believed to have a role.
• Disturbances of neurotransmitter release, whether of endogenous (e.g. in disorders of brain function) or exogenous origin (e.g. by drugs), are likely therefore to affect food intake.

Drugs that affect release of neurotransmitters (e.g. serotonin reuptake inhibitors) are used to help in weight loss. However, other drugs that are prescribed for the treatment of mental illness may have an effect on neurotransmitters involved in food intake, and thereby cause increases or decreases in food consumption.

Role of diet in behaviour and disease

The role of diet in the function of the brain, and in everyday behaviour, disordered behaviour and disease is of great interest. Research into these links is ongoing; some areas are summarised in Table 36.1.

Much work is still needed on the nutritional needs of normal brain function; such studies are complicated by the ethical issues involved and the complexity of human behaviour.

Eating disorders

In disordered eating, food intake patterns may appear to be outside the rational control of the subject, and may be seen as part of a mental health disorder.

Most generally, there may be a preoccupation with slimming diets, or fad eating, which coexists with restrained eating, and is associated with a 'fear of fatness'.

Recognised eating disorders may form a continuum, from the most restricted eating, as seen in anorexia nervosa, through binge-purge behaviour, as seen in bulimia nervosa, to binge eating characterising some cases of obesity (see Figure 36.1). Specific diagnostic criteria exist for the better recognised conditions of anorexia nervosa and bulimia nervosa.

Anorexia nervosa

This represents the most severe deficit, with extremely low energy intakes over a period of time, resulting in weight loss. Energy intake may be further reduced by self-induced vomiting and use of laxatives. Weight loss may be accelerated by high levels of energy expenditure. Micronutrient status is also likely to be poor, although requirements may be reduced. Consequently, there are physiological changes typical of starvation, which affect all systems of the body. Most notable are changes to:

• gastrointestinal tract (poor motility, delayed gastric emptying, bloating, constipation, anatomical damage due to vomiting and overeating in binges);
• musculoskeletal system (loss of muscle and demineralisation of bone);
• endocrine system (depressed activity of reproductive system

Table 36.1 Some suggested dietary links with brain function.

Behaviour/disease state	Suggested dietary links/evidence
Mood	Evidence suggests that carbohydrate intake may elevate mood, due to increases in brain serotonin levels Carbohydrate 'craving' and 'addiction' described, but evidence is equivocal
Stress-induced eating	Associated with higher intakes of either protein-rich or carbohydrate-rich foods May be related to release of catecholamines, or levels of sex hormones in women during phases of menstrual cycle
Depression	Possibly related to low levels of n-3 fatty acids in the diet; some supplementation trials have shown benefits, but evidence still equivocal Folate, iron and selenium status have all been linked with depression
Attention-deficit hyperactivity disorder (ADHD)	Relationship with n-3/n-6 fatty acid imbalance suggested More trials needed
Autism	Some suggestions of a link with gluten sensitivity; more evidence needed
Alzheimer's disease/ other dementias	Current evidence suggests a link with raised homocysteine levels. Also link with antioxidant status However, results from supplementation trials with B vitamins or antioxidant nutrients have failed to replicate epidemiological findings High levels of some metals, e.g. iron, copper, zinc, aluminium, have been proposed as contributing to oxidative damage
Disruptive/antisocial behaviour	Trials on prisoners and offenders have suggested that an improvement in overall nutritional intake, by removal of refined carbohydrates and inclusion of more balanced nutrient-rich meals, is rapidly followed by less antisocial behaviour Such studies have also been performed in schools, using mineral and vitamin supplements, in which increases in IQ were reported. Further work is needed

hormones, high levels of cortisol, low levels of thyroid hormones – leading to low metabolic rate and hypothermia);

• central nervous system (may have poor memory and concentration, depression, irritability, some evidence of reduction in brain substance);

• cardiovascular system (reduction in size of heart, lower blood pressure, poor circulation to periphery, cardiac arrhythmias);

• blood (fewer red and white blood cells, reduced immunity).

The condition is characterised by a disturbed body image and any treatment requires a multifactorial approach addressing both the requirements for food as well as the underlying psychological causes.

Bulimia nervosa

This is characterised by episodes of binge eating, during which energy intakes are very high, averaging at least 2000 kcal. These are generally accompanied by the use of laxatives, diuretics and self-induced vomiting. The episodes are triggered by 'loss of control' in the majority of cases. There may also be excessive exercising and strict dieting between these episodes. Body weight may be in the normal range, and the typical features of starvation absent. Food intakes may be relatively normal outside binge episodes.

The bingeing, vomiting and purging result in damage to the gut, teeth and salivary glands, as well as causing electrolyte imbalances (especially of potassium) and the risk of dehydration. Other minerals affected include calcium, magnesium, phosphate and sodium.

Kidney damage has been reported from overuse of diuretics.

Binge eating disorder may be differentiated from bulimia nervosa as it lacks the compensatory energy dissipating mechanisms. It is therefore more likely to be associated with obesity, and thus the accompanying health problems.

As with anorexia nervosa, treatment of both bulimia nervosa and binge eating requires behavioural approaches.

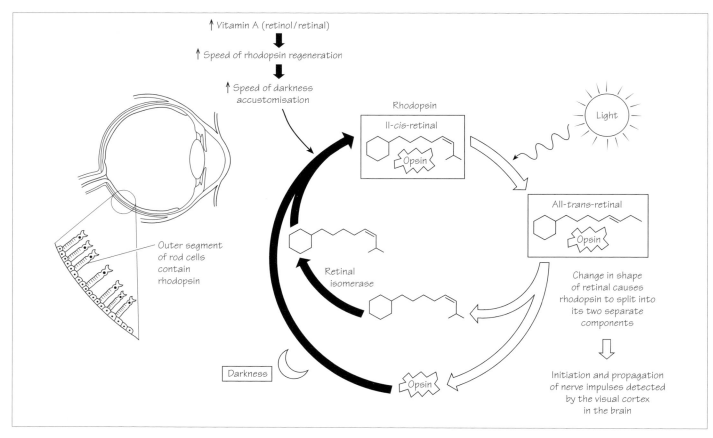

Fig. 37.1 Role of vitamin A in vision (reproduced with permission from Barasi, M. (2003) *Human Nutrition: A Health Perspective*, Hodder Arnold).

Aims

(1) To describe the role of nutrition in the structure and function of the eye.
(2) To consider the consequences of nutritional deficiencies on eye function.

The eye as a sensory receptor provides visual information enabling us to obtain and enjoy food. The visual appeal of foods is important to encourage consumption. Individuals who have visual impairment are potentially disadvantaged in terms of their ability to control their food intake.

Adequate nutrient supplies are vital for the eye during development and in maintaining its integrity and function, and a loss of function in older age may be caused by a failing supply of protective nutrients.

Structure of the eye: introduction to nutritional links

The essential light-sensitive area of the eye is the *retina,* containing *rods* (about 100 million) and *cones* (about 3 million); it lines the interior of the inner eye. The eye is supported by the choroid, which supplies nutrients via the blood. The sclera encases the inner eye, and rests within a fat-lined socket, supported by muscles that allow the eye to move.

Thiamin deficiency may cause paralysis of these muscles and affect eye movement. The fat provides a supportive cushion and loss of this fat in **starvation** may result in potential damage to the eye on impact.

Retinal function and nutrition

In both the rods and cones the opsin proteins are associated with 11-*cis*-retinal, derived from retinol. Rhodopsin, found in the rods, is more sensitive to a lack of retinol than is iodopsin, the pigment in the cones.

The sequence of events in the photosensitive cells of the retina is shown in Figure 37.1.

The time taken for rhodopsin to be sufficiently resynthesised for vision to be possible in dim light is known as the *dark adaptation time.* Individuals who are vitamin A deficient have poor dark adaptation and may be unable to see clearly in the dark.

Optic nerve neuropathy

A deficiency of **vitamin B$_{12}$**, occurring in individuals infested with fish tapeworm, and in heavy smokers and drinkers, has been reported as causing demyelination of the optic nerve and impaired vision. Cyanide toxicity, generated from cassava-based diets, may also cause

Potential problems with the retinal cycle

- Retinol-binding protein is required to transport retinol to the eye; *poor protein status* will affect the formation of rhodopsin.
- *A low-fat diet* may reduce the absorption of vitamin A.
- *Zinc deficiency* will compromise the visual cycle, as it is required for the synthesis of opsin and the conversion of retinol to retinal.
- The rods contain high levels of docosahexaenoic acid (DHA), an *n*-3 fatty acid, which provides them with flexibility, and contributes to their role in vision. Visual acuity is reported to be affected when diets *lack n-3 fatty acids* during key developmental stages.
- The retina contains substantial amounts of the amino acid *taurine*, which stabilises the cell membranes. Requirements are high in the newborn. Both taurine and *n*-3 fatty acids are present in greater amounts in human milk than in formula milk, although some milks are now fortified with both.

damage to the optic nerve in situations where B_{12} is deficient, as this would normally limit the toxic effects of cyanide.

The macula

High levels of *carotenoid pigments*, such as zeaxanthin and lutein, are found in the macula.

- It is believed that they provide powerful *antioxidant protection* against the effects of reactive oxygen species generated by light entering the eye, which is focused at this area for central vision.
- There is also a very high oxygen tension within the retina, contributing to potential oxidative damage.

Retinopathy

Premature infants who are treated with hyperbaric oxygen may experience degeneration of retinal arteries, or retinopathy of prematurity. This has been associated with *deficiency of vitamin E*, and supplements may be protective to an extent.

Age-related macular degeneration (ARMD)

In this condition, abnormal material is deposited within the macula, between the retina and the choroid. This leads to gradual loss of central vision and ability to perceive fine detail.

It is the *leading cause of registered blindness* in Western populations, and increases with age.

Maintaining adequate intakes of antioxidants, particularly those carotenoids found in the macula, may prevent or delay the onset of ARMD. The condition is particularly common in smokers, whose intakes of lutein are lower than the population average.

Lutein cannot be synthesised by the body, so a dietary intake is required. Breast milk, green leafy vegetables and orange/yellow fruits and vegetables are good sources.

Retinopathy may also occur as a result of damage to blood vessels supplying the retina. This can be the consequence of *hypertension*, or of deposition of glycated proteins in capillary walls in *diabetes*. The latter causes thickening and destruction of the capillaries, leading to blurring of vision. Diabetic retinopathy is more likely the longer the duration of diabetes, and with poorer control.

The retina may also be damaged by *glaucoma*, which is an increased pressure within the eyeball that ultimately damages the optic nerve. This may also lead to ARMD and cataract formation.

The lens and nutrition

Cataracts are the result of an increased opacity of the lens, often accompanied by loss of accommodation. The lens is exposed to ultraviolet light and oxidising products.

- Glutathione and glutathione reductase, which act as *antioxidants*, are present in high concentrations, but levels decline with age.
- Levels of reduced glutathione are maintained by *niacin, riboflavin* and *vitamin C*.
- Cataracts are more common in lower income groups, smokers and those exposed to more direct sunlight; protection against antioxidant damage appears to be important.

The cornea and conjunctiva

The front of the eye is exposed to the external environment and requires effective protection. The conjunctiva is lubricated by the tears secreted by the lacrimal glands.

The integrity of the conjunctiva is dependent on normal epithelial cell differentiation to maintain barrier function and mucus secretion. These require adequate *vitamin A* status, and deficiency results in *xerophthalmia*, or dry eye. There is a failure of tear production and the eye lacks lysozyme to keep it clean. It becomes susceptible to bacterial infections, resulting in conjunctivitis and ultimately infection of the cornea, which becomes ulcerated and keratinised. If untreated the condition leads to *keratomalacia,* with permanent scarring of the eyeball and blindness.

Zinc is concentrated in the cornea and deficiency may result in corneal oedema, conjunctivitis and xerosis.

Deficiency of *riboflavin* results in blockage of the sebaceous glands of the eyelids, which become inflamed and painful. There is also photophobia and excessive tear production, and new blood vessels may be produced on the cornea. Lens opacity may increase. Riboflavin is believed to be important in facilitating oxygen supply to the front of the eye.

Wilson's disease, a genetic defect of *copper* metabolism, results in characteristic deposition of copper in the cornea (Kayser–Fleischer rings). Chelating drugs may be used in this condition to excrete excess copper from the body.

In familial *hypercholesterolaemia*, deposits of cholesterol are characteristic within the cornea.

The health of the eye thus requires good nutrition for its function, but may also reflect the state of health of the individual, as more general deficiencies or excesses are evident in the appearance of this organ.

38 Nutrition in pregnancy and lactation

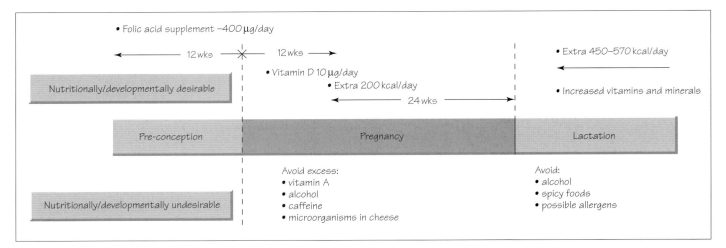

Fig. 38.1 A summary of desirable and undesirable nutritional practices in pregnancy and lactation.

Aims

(1) To describe the nutritional needs of pregnancy and lactation.
(2) To identify nutritional advice for pregnancy and lactation.

In terms of physiological processes, preparation for pregnancy and lactation occurs during growth and development. Nutritional status will influence the capacity to support the pregnancy to a successful outcome.

Nutrition at conception

Nutritional status at the time of conception is critical in early fetal development.

Fertility is affected by *body weight*, and is at its optimum at the normal BMI range of 20–25.
• In women with BMI <18 there may be amenorrhoea, and ovulatory failure.
• In obese women, there may also be polycystic ovary syndrome (PCOS), resulting in ovulatory failure.
• A high waist to hip ratio (>0.8) is associated with lower fertility. Weight normalisation is frequently all that is needed to help infertile women to conceive.

Supplementation with folic acid during the period around conception can reduce the incidence of neural tube defects (NTD). It is now recommended that all girls and women who may become pregnant supplement with 400 µg/day of folic acid, from at least 3 months before conception until 12 weeks of pregnancy. This intake can only be met from supplements, as dietary sources do not contain such high, or bioavailable levels.

Mainly because at least 50% of pregnancies are unplanned, the correct uptake of folic acid supplements in the UK is low. Some countries (e.g. USA, Canada) now add folic acid to flour, and NTD rates have fallen substantially there. There is a proposal in the UK to fortify flour with folic acid.

Adequate nutrient stores are vital to sustain implantation and organ formation in the first weeks of pregnancy, as the placenta is not fully functional until the third month of pregnancy, to act as a 'nutritional gatekeeper' for the fetus.

Nutrition during pregnancy

Several adaptations occur in the mother's body to increase the efficiency of nutrient provision.

Energy needs and weight gain

The typical increase in weight (in the UK) during pregnancy is 11–16 kg but varies widely. Gains in the second and third trimesters should average 0.4 kg/week for normal weight women, less (0.3 kg/week) for overweight women and more (0.5 kg/week) for women who are underweight.
• Excessive weight gain is associated with a large baby, increases the risk of complications at delivery, and should be managed by dietary advice. Reducing diets are not recommended.
• Low weight gain carries the risk of a low-birth-weight baby, with possible long-term health implications.

The extra energy costs of pregnancy are estimated at 310 MJ (77 000 kcal). Adjustments occur to the mother's metabolic rate to increase efficiency of energy use.

Advice for women planning to conceive
- Avoidance of excessive vitamin A (retinol) (especially in liver and liver products) – potential teratogenic effect.
- Avoidance of binge drinking – teratogenic effect.
- Reduction in smoking (to zero if possible).
- Avoidance of excessive amounts of caffeine (>300 mg/day).
- Avoidance of foods that may contain microorganisms, such as unpasteurised milk or cheese.
- A balanced healthy diet, including fruit and vegetables, to provide micronutrients, sufficient iron intake and fish consumption to provide PUFAs.

Many women achieve energy savings by reducing their activity, and increasing their food intake by a small amount.

In general it is better to monitor weight gain rather than precisely specifying energy needs. However, in the UK, an additional (0.8 MJ) 200 kcal/day is recommended in the last trimester.

Iron needs

Expansion of the blood volume requires additional iron. Iron can be provided from:
- Body stores (up to 50% of women may have low or no stores).
- Cessation of menstruation.
- Increase in iron absorption in the gut.
- Iron supplements.
- Dietary intake (see Table 38.1).

Calcium needs

Calcium requirements are increased in the last trimester of pregnancy.

Calcium is provided from:
- Remodelling of the bone, facilitated by oestrogen, prolactin and increased levels of active vitamin D.
- Increased absorption.

Vitamin D levels must be adequate; advice is to take a vitamin D supplement to achieve an intake of 10 μg/day, especially in winter pregnancies, or when skin is regularly covered for cultural reasons.

In teenage pregnancies, extra requirements should be met with increased intake of rich sources such as milk, dairy products, nuts, pulses, bread and tinned fish.

Calcium is also important for the maintenance of normal blood pressure in pregnancy.

Other nutrients

- *Long-chain PUFAs* are needed for development of the brain and retina. Sources are oily fish; some can be synthesised from α-linolenic acid, found in oils (soya, rapeseed and walnut), green vegetables and meat from grass-fed animals.

- Requirements of *protein* and *B vitamins* (except folate) increase in line with energy needs. Therefore women eating to appetite from a balanced diet, should meet these requirements.
- *Iron, potassium, magnesium, calcium, iodine, vitamin A* and *riboflavin* have been found to be low in some diets in pregnant women.

At-risk groups

Special attention is needed for nutrition in some groups of women (Table 38.2).

Lactation

The mother's nutritional status is unlikely to affect the volume or the macronutrient content of her milk for the first few weeks of lactation. However, poorly nourished women will not be able to sustain the same level of nutrients for prolonged periods.

The fat content of the milk correlates with the mother's levels of body fat, and the pattern of fatty acids secreted in the milk partly reflects those in the mother's dietary intake.

Neither the fat-soluble vitamin content nor the mineral content of the milk fluctuates with maternal dietary intake.

The levels of water-soluble vitamins will vary, depending on intakes, and therefore supplementation of the mother will be reflected by raised levels in her milk.

Women who are vegetarian or vegan may need additional supplementation with vitamin B_{12}, vitamin D (if there is insufficient sunlight exposure) and calcium.

Potentially harmful substances, such as alcohol, drugs and allergens, that may pass through the milk should be avoided.

Although human milk is the ideal food for almost all babies, many women in westernised countries choose not to breast feed. Health promotion and education information about breast feeding has caused some increase in breast-feeding rates in the UK, but levels still lag behind those in other European countries.

Recommendations for lactation
- An additional 1.9–2.4 MJ (450–570 kcal)/day, depending on stage of lactation.
- Increase in nutrients related to energy intakes (protein and B vitamins).
- Increase in nutrients secreted in substantial amounts in the milk: calcium, phosphorus, magnesium and zinc, folate, vitamin A and C.

Table 38.1 Practical advice on iron intakes.

Useful sources of iron	Factors that improve iron absorption
Lean red meat, eggs	Sources of vitamin C with meals
Pulses, dark-green leafy vegetables	Avoid tea/coffee with meals
Bread, fortified breakfast cereals	Eating animal sources of iron improves
Dried fruit	absorption from plant sources

Table 38.2 Population groups who may be at risk of not meeting nutritional needs in pregnancy.

Group	Reasons for risk	Action/advice
Teenagers	Own needs for growth still high	Ensure high dietary quality
	May deny pregnancy, be reluctant to adjust diet/behaviour	Focus on adequate weight gain, calcium, iron and folate intakes
Overweight/ obese	Increased risk of complications, including preterm delivery, hypertension, gestational diabetes (GDM)	Keep gain within recommended levels Ensure dietary quality, advise exercise Use slowly absorbed carbohydrates and regular meals to manage GDM
Vegetarian/ vegan	Potential for lower nutrient intakes	Ensure balanced/varied diet to provide a range of micronutrients Long-chain PUFAs, iron, zinc, calcium and vitamin D may be particular issues
Low income	Poorer reserves at start of pregnancy, lower micronutrient intakes, less weight gain, higher risk of low birth weight	Advise on cheaper sources of nutrient-rich foods, such as fortified breakfast cereals, bread, tinned pulses, fruit and vegetables, small amounts of meat, tinned fish

Nutrition in infants and preschool children

Aims

(1) To describe the nutritional content of human and formula milk in relation to the nutritional needs of infants.

(2) To explain the process of complementary feeding (weaning) of infants.

(3) To consider the nutritional needs of preschool children.

The challenge in meeting nutritional needs in infants arises from:

- *limited capacity for food* due to the infant's size and immaturity of the digestive and excretory systems;
- *relatively high demand for nutrients* to fulfil the needs for growth;
- *total dependence* on another person for the provision of food.

Growth rates

The fastest rate of growth is in the first 6 months of life, with a doubling of birth weight, and slows towards 12 months, to achieve about three times birth weight. Body weight only doubles between the ages of 1 and 5 years.

Standard growth charts are useful to check that growth is progressing appropriately; rates that rise too steeply or fall below the expected trajectory need attention and explanation.

The optimum food for an infant is human breast milk, and this is the reference for both nutrient requirement values for this age group and any alternative milk formulae.

Breast feeding

The composition of breast milk ensures that it is readily digested and absorbed (Table 39.1).

Other benefits of breast feeding

Apart from the nutritional advantages, there are other benefits of breast feeding for both the mother and infant.

- For the infant, there is less risk of infection, especially gastrointestinal and respiratory infection, and improved cognitive development.
- For the mother, there is a period of anovulation (which may help with birth spacing) and reduced risk of premenopausal breast cancer.

Table 39.1 Factors in breast milk facilitating digestion and absorption.

Factor	Effect on digestion and absorption
High lactose content	Promotes calcium absorption Supplies galactose for brain development
High whey protein content	More readily digested than casein
Non-protein nitrogen	Includes taurine, urea and growth factors, which may be utilised in the colon
Lipids profile	Contains lipase and bile salts to facilitate fat digestion
Specific binding proteins for vitamins and minerals	Facilitate absorption, prevent their use by microorganisms

In addition, human milk contains *protective factors* that are critical in the early weeks of an infant's life when its own defences are undeveloped (Table 39.2).

Nutritional content of breast milk

The actual composition of breast milk (Table 39.3) varies between mothers, between feeds and during a feed in the same mother.

Formula milk

Infant formula, designed to meet the complete nutritional needs of infants up to 4–6 months of age, is subject to strict regulations, via EC directives and government regulations.

Formula milk is derived from cow's milk, and is classified as:

- 'casein dominated' when based on the entire protein fraction, or
- 'whey dominated', containing the dialysed whey protein.

Further modifications include the addition of lactose, maltodextrins, vegetable oils, trace elements and vitamins, and reduction in the levels of electrolytes, calcium and phosphorus. Some manufacturers add long-chain fatty acids, taurine and carnitine.

For infants who are allergic to components of milk, soya-derived formula is available. In addition there are formulae available for low-birth-weight and preterm babies.

'Follow-on' milks are also available for use beyond the age of 6 months; these are modified (e.g. with extra iron) and as such are better than cow's milk, but there is little evidence that they are superior to the continued use of ordinary formula, together with complementary feeding, which should have been started.

Complementary feeding (weaning)

The WHO has concluded that breast feeding should remain exclusive to the age of 6 months and that complementary feeding should be started at this time. This policy has also been adopted in the UK, where it is also recommended that foods other than milk should not be introduced before the age of 4 months.

To achieve normal developmental goals, suitable foods need to be introduced at an appropriate pace to match the infant's capabilities.

- Introduction too early may give rise to allergic reactions due to

Table 39.2 Protective factors occurring in human milk.

Protective factor	Function	Additional information
Secretory immunoglobulin A	Protects mucosal surface against antigens Primes immune system	The IgA is thought to be primed to react to antigens to which the mother is exposed
Macrophages, lymphocytes, lysozyme	Engulf bacteria; secrete immunoglobulins and lymphokines	General defence against infective organisms
Lactoferrin	Binds iron	Competes with bacteria for iron, restricting their growth
Bifidus factor	Stimulates growth of bifidobacteria and lactobacilli, reducing the pH	Aided by the presence of nonabsorbed oligosaccharides and residual lactose, which provide a food source

Table 39.3 Macronutrient composition of mature human milk compared with whey-dominated infant formula (values are per litre of milk).

Nutrient	Human milk	Infant formula
Energy MJ (kcal)	2.95 (700)	2.8 (670)
Protein (g)	11–13[a]	15
Fat (g)	42–45	36
Carbohydrate (g)	70	72

[a]There is a great deal of uncertainty about the actual protein content of human milk.

Reasons for introducing additional foods

- Provision of more energy and nutrients to meet growth needs.
- Provision of iron, as supplies from birth become depleted.
- Developmental stimulation: hand to mouth, facial and oral developments, essential for speech.
- Able to cope with digestion, absorption and excretion of other foods.
- Development of social skills, eating with the family.
- Acquisition of taste discrimination.

A suggested scheme for progressive weaning

Stage 1
Smooth puree (generally as single item): e.g. non-wheat cereal (to avoid development of gluten allergy), puréed cooked vegetables, dairy products.

Stage 2
Mashed and lumpy food: e.g. minced meat, fish, cheese, vegetables and fruit.

Stage 3
Finger food (from about 7 months): e.g. rusks, fingers of toast, pieces of hard cheese, fruit or vegetable.

Drink in a cup to be introduced as suckling declines: milk, water, very diluted fruit juice.

the immaturity of the gut, and possibly be associated with more chest infections and obesity.

- Delayed introduction may miss the developmental 'window' when the ability to chew first occurs, and result in growth faltering due to insufficient nutrition.

Throughout weaning:
- An infant may take some *time* to become accustomed to new

Intake at 12 months

A day's intake may include three meals and three snacks, including the following:

- Cereal foods – four portions
- Fruit and vegetables – four portions
- Milk group – two portions, +350 mL milk, or equivalent
- Meat or alternatives – two portions

flavours and textures, so new foods need to be tried several times.
- Feeding should always be *supervised* to avoid danger of choking.
- Foods containing *iron* and *calcium* should always be included.
- A low-fat or high-fibre diet is not appropriate.
- *Salt* and *sugar* should *not* be added to food.
- Nuts (choking) and honey (microbial contamination) should not be given.
- Soft-boiled eggs, paté and mould-ripened cheese should also be avoided (contamination risk).
- *Energy density* of the foods should meet energy and nutrient requirements. Commercially prepared foods can be more nutrient dense than homemade meals.

Supplementary vitamin drops, containing vitamins A, C and D, are recommended for all children under 2 years in the UK. Breast-fed children should receive these from the age of 6 months; those receiving formula do not require these until transfer to cow's milk at 12 months.

A child following its growth centile and developing a broad appetite for various foods is a good indicator of successful weaning.

Preschool children

Between the age of 1 and 5 years a child moves from a diet dependent on milk for many nutrients and containing up to 50% of its energy as fat, towards one that meets the dietary guidelines and contains items from all food groups. Family food should form the basis of the diet (Table 39.4).

Children in this age group may be looked after by parents, but an increasing number may attend day-care facilities, where they receive food. Guidelines exist for provision of healthy food for snacks and lunch in nursery or day care units.

Nutritional principles to be addressed include:
- Achieving the DRVs for this age group.
- Low-fat diets are not recommended.
- Attention to nutrient density – especially at risk are calcium, iron, zinc, vitamin A and vitamin C.
- Avoidance of excess amounts of non-milk extrinsic sugar or fatty foods.

Table 39.4 Some issues that may arise in preschool children.

Issue	Possible strategy/advice
Food refusal, fussy eating, narrow range of foods eaten	Parents/carers to provide example, eat with family, introduce foods gradually, keep trying with new foods, do not offer a range of alternatives for disliked foods
'Grazing' between meals – limits appetite at mealtimes	Restrict between-meal food availability; eating is an 'event' and not a passive accompaniment to other activities
High consumption of fruit juice and soft drinks	Risk of effect on appetite and dental health: offer only water, diluted fruit juice. Soft drinks occasionally only
Low-fat/high-fibre diet perceived by parents as 'healthy'	Ensure child is able to consume sufficient to meet needs; growth pattern critical. Low-fat products inappropriate before age of 2 years. Gradually increase wholefoods during this period, as appetite allows
High level of snack food consumption – cakes, biscuits, crisps, confectionery, sweets	Offer alternative snacks – fruit, scones, yogurt, toast + spread, plain popcorn, dry breakfast cereal
Foods used as rewards	Use alternative rewards, not food related

Nutrition in school-age children and adolescents

Aims
(1) To describe nutritional needs during childhood and adolescence.
(2) To consider how these needs can be met and the problems that may arise.

Growth rates
Growth and development occur over a long period in humans, from conception to late adolescence. During the years of childhood, mean growth is relatively constant, and averages 2.5 kg and 6 cm per year. During puberty, on average:
- girls increase by 20 cm (height) and 20 kg (weight);
- boys increase by 30 cm (height) and 30 kg (weight).

These increases represent 40% of eventual adult weight.

Growth is vulnerable to faltering if nutritional intakes do not keep pace with the demands.

Body composition
- Body fat percentage levels increase rapidly in the first months of life, but start to fall after the first year.
- There is a further increase from about the age of 5 years (adiposity rebound), which may start earlier in larger, fatter children, and could be associated with higher risk of later nutrition-related non-communicable diseases (NR-NCDs). In boys, the fat content starts to fall during the pubertal growth spurt, but in girls it continues to increase, resulting in the average 10% fat content differential between the sexes seen in adults.
- A critical fat mass is essential for menarche in girls; leptin is proposed as the link between nutritional status and the initiation of menstruation.
- Lean body mass increases throughout childhood, but particularly in males during puberty.
- Changes in height require bone growth to be maintained, and as weight increases at puberty, the bones increase in strength with their most rapid period of mineral accretion.

Nutritional needs
Dietary recommendations reflect the change in body size and composition. During childhood, nutritional needs for the majority of nutrients are the same for boys and girls, and increase only slightly between the younger (4–6) and older (7–10) years.

Once into adolescence, there are much greater demands, reflected in increased recommended levels, which should be met by increased intakes from all food groups (Table 40.1).

The diet should provide:
- sources of starchy carbohydrates – five servings per day;
- fruit and vegetables – five servings per day;
- milk and dairy products – three servings per day;
- meat and alternatives – two servings per day.

Fatty and sugary foods should be limited in the diet, and only consumed when the other groups have been adequately provided. Attention to variety reduces the risk of omitting particular nutrients.

Data collected in surveys of young people aged 4–18 years suggest that diets are not in line with recommendations (see Tables 40.2 and 40.3).

Additional influences that may have health consequences are considered in Chapter 41.

School meals
In school, food needs to be provided for children to:
- sustain their ability to concentrate and learn;
- make a contribution to overall dietary intake;
- teach about food and nutrition, as well as social aspects of eating.

In recent years, children in the UK have been choosing to eat chips, burgers and other high-fat main dishes, cakes and soft drinks, with few selecting fruit, vegetables or salads. As a result the nutritional quality of school meals has been criticised for having:
- too much fat, supplying 41% of the energy in the meal (recommended level is 35%);
- too much saturated fat, supplying 14% of energy (recommended 11%);

Table 40.1 Main nutritional needs in adolescence.

Nutrient	Reason for increased need	Additional points to note
Energy	Synthesis of new tissue is energy demanding. Increased body size results in an increase in metabolic rate, and energy needs for activity	Needs are greater in boys than girls, linked to larger overall size
Protein	Synthesis of new tissues	Intakes generally high in UK. Restricted diets (see below) may be inadequate
Fats	Unsaturated fatty acids needed for membranes. Cholesterol synthesis increases for synthesis of sex hormones	Diets containing large amounts of 'fast foods' may not contain sufficient unsaturated fats
B vitamins	Cofactors for metabolic and synthetic reactions	Needs increase in line with energy (for thiamin and niacin) and protein (pyridoxine)
Iron, copper, folate and vitamin B_{12}	Required for expansion of blood cell mass to support extra tissues. In girls onset of menstruation increases iron requirements	Poor iron status may result in impairment of cognitive function
Calcium and vitamin D	Needed for skeletal growth	Additional nutrients also required for the skeleton include: vitamins A, C and K, and phosphorus, magnesium, potassium and zinc

Table 40.2 Some findings relating to diets of adolescents in the UK.

Positive features of diets	Negative features of diets
Cereals and cereal products are main source of energy	Cereal products also contribute to fat intakes
Milk consumed most by the youngest groups	Carbonated drinks commonly drunk by oldest groups
Protein intakes adequate: children taller and heavier than earlier cohorts	Non-milk extrinsic sugars provide 16.5% of energy (recommended 10%)
Fruit popular with younger children, consumption decreases sharply with age	Green vegetables consumed by fewer than 50%; raw and salad vegetables consumed by about 50%
Most micronutrient intakes above Reference Nutrient Intake (RNI), for most age groups	Risk of micronutrient intakes below LRNI in older children Specifically: all vitamins in older girls, iron (50% of oldest girls), calcium, potassium (15% of oldest boys), magnesium (18% of oldest boys), zinc and iodine

Table 40.3 Factors influencing nutritional intakes in adolescents in the UK.

Factor	Consequence
Independence	Own food choices, linked to availability of money, rejection of parental influences
Growth	Large variation in appetite, as growth rates vary
Illness and infection	Exposure to other children in school leads to infections and loss of appetite during illness
Activity	May become sedentary in adolescence
Peer pressure	Can cause significant changes in eating habits; may start smoking (increases needs for antioxidants), drinking alcohol (may displace nutrient-dense foods and affect absorption of folate, thiamin, vitamin C and calcium)
Advertising	Fatty and sugary foods promoted

- too much non-milk extrinsic sugar, supplying 14% of energy (recommended 11%);
- too much salt;
- too few fruit and vegetables.

New initiatives

In order to improve children's diets in UK schools, a variety of *means to engage all the major participants* in meal provision have been developed:
- creation of new standards for school meals, with food- and nutrient-based guidelines (see Table 40.4);
- engagement of parents, schools and local authorities;
- restriction on certain foods and drinks within schools;
- improving school kitchens and upgrading training and qualifications for catering staff;
- inclusion of school food provision as part of the school inspection process.

Table 40.4 Summary of revised Caroline Walker Trust guidelines for school meals, introduced from 2006.

Nutrient	Guideline
Energy	30% of the estimated average requirement (EAR) for energy
Fat	Total fat: not more than 35% of food energy SFAs: not more than 11% of food energy
Carbohydrate	Not more than 50% of food energy
Non-milk extrinsic sugars	Not more than 11% of food energy
Fibre	Not less than 30% of calculated reference value (based on 18 g for adults)
Protein	Not less than 30% of the RNI
Iron, zinc, calcium	Not less than 40% of RNI
Vitamin A, vitamin C, folate	Not less than 40% of RNI
Sodium/salt	Not more than 30% of the SACN target
Fruit and vegetables	Not less than two portions
Oily fish	On menu at least once per week
Fried/processed potato products	Not on menu more than once per week

Also included is:
- advice on additional meal provision within the school, such as breakfast and after-school clubs;
- advice for parents on the content of packed lunches.

Other targets for improvement include: tuck shops, vending machines, dining room environments and provision of water.

Initiatives to encourage children's involvement with food include growing food in school allotments, and cookery clubs.

By both enhancing the interest in food, and improving the variety and quality of food provided in school, the aim is to reverse some of the deterioration in the dietary habits of school children, and ultimately halt the increase in obesity and associated health problems.

41

Nutritional problems in infants, children and adolescents

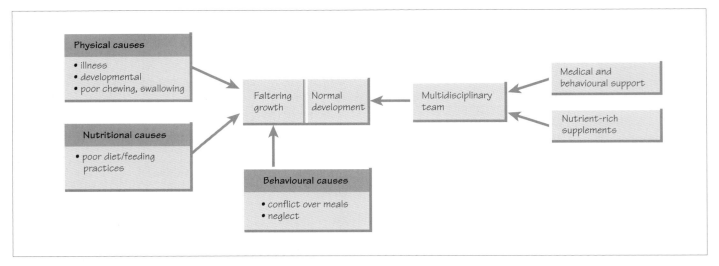

Fig. 41.1 Factors leading to faltering growth in infants, and remedial actions.

Aims

(1) To describe some issues associated with poor nutrition in children.

(2) To identify some practices that may lead to poor nutritional status. These age groups are vulnerable because:

- nutritional needs relative to their size are greater than in adulthood;
- there is a smaller margin for error with nutritional intakes.

Low birth weight

Low birth weight (LBW; <2500 g) may arise because the baby:

- is born preterm;
- has suffered intrauterine growth retardation (IUGR) and is small for gestational age (SGA).

Such infants have high nutritional requirements, but limited capacity and developmental ability to cope with normal nutrition. Feeding is via nasogastric tube where possible, until sucking and swallowing reflexes are sufficiently developed for bottle or breast feeding.

Feeding LBW babies

(1) Mothers who deliver prematurely produce *breast milk* with a higher energy and protein content than term milk, and this is highly beneficial for the infant, in nutritional, immunological and developmental terms. It is better tolerated with easier establishment of feeding, and reduced risks of complications. Later, there are higher developmental scores.

(2) *Expressed breast milk* may be enhanced with breast milk fortifiers (BMF) to boost some nutrient levels.

(3) If breast milk is not available, *preterm formula* may be used, which is more nutrient dense than normal formula milks, containing more energy, protein and minerals. Vitamin supplements, including vitamins A, C, D and folic acid, may also be needed. Iron supplements are generally not given as these may act as a pro-oxidant.

(4) Very small babies may need to be fed via the intravenous route, but enteral feeding is started as soon as possible.

Growth faltering

Growth in infants and young children, usually recorded as weight, should progress along a centile line on standard growth charts. Reasons for centile crossing (moving from one centile line to another) need to be established.

- Infants of diabetic mothers, who are often born very large (>4.5 kg), may exhibit 'catch-down' growth during the first year of life. Once removed from the oversupply of nutrients in the womb, their growth rate slows.
- An infant undernourished in the womb may show 'catch-up' growth. This should be an increase in lean body mass, rather than fat; the latter is linked to risk of later disease.

Other reasons for growth faltering are summarised in Figure 41.1.

With appropriate intervention, a child should exhibit 'catch-up' growth and return to its growth centile.

Overweight and obesity

The prevalence of overweight and obesity has been increasing rapidly among children around the world in line with the general trend of increasing obesity across all ages.

A definition of overweight and obesity in children is difficult, because body mass index (BMI) changes throughout this period, and standard adult 'cut-off' values cannot be used.

However, the *likely attainment* of an adult BMI above 25 or 30 can be projected from existing data, and superimposed on BMI charts for children and adolescents as indicators of future risk.

The *causes* of this increase are multifactorial, but are likely to include:

- a reduced level of physical activity (more sedentary leisure activities, less effort used in daily travel, reduced open play space, poor quality environments);
- passive overconsumption as a result of increased snacking on energy-dense foods and drinks, a process fuelled by advertising;

- reduced consumption of freshly prepared meals, following the trend towards manufactured and processed foods, containing more energy per unit weight;
- increased availability of these foods.

Preventing/managing excess weight gain

Avoidance of excess weight gain and early intervention in overweight are key aspects for health professionals (Table 41.1). Allowing the child to 'grow into' a more appropriate weight for his or her age is a practical solution. Common approaches include:
- Reducing energy intake:
  - foods with high satiety value
  - regular meals
  - reduce snacks/drinks with 'empty calories'
  - involvement with food selection and preparation;
- Increasing energy output:
  - encourage movement
  - reduce sedentary pastimes
  - involve family in activity.

Iron status

Iron deficiency anaemia affects about 9% of young children and adolescents in the UK. Many more have low stores and poor iron status; up to half of adolescent girls have intakes well below recommendations.

Advice on sources of dietary iron that are acceptable in this age group is needed. Iron supplements may be recommended if dietary intakes cannot be increased.

Teenage girls need adequate iron stores in anticipation of childbearing needs when they reach adulthood.

Vegetarianism

Exclusion of animal foods from the diet is reported by 5% of the UK population. Vegetarian diets may be introduced to children by their parents; as children become more independent, and especially in adolescence, they may choose for themselves to become vegetarian.

A well-balanced vegetarian diet can provide all the necessary nutrients for growth and development. But if there is insufficient

Causes of low iron status
- Reserves present at birth are depleted by 4–6 months; iron must be supplied in the weaning diet.
- In the first year, diets that exclude meat and fortified cereals or formula milk may lead to poor iron status.
- Fussy eaters are vulnerable. Carers may need advice on enhancing iron absorption.
- Needs remain high throughout growth, to form haemoglobin, iron-containing enzymes and for menstruation from puberty.

Consequences of low iron status
- Anaemia, characterised by pallor, tiredness, apathy, breathlessness and poor appetite, poor growth.
- Effects on cognitive development, poor attention span and lack of interest in learning, limited achievement in school.

knowledge or planning to select a balanced intake, deficiencies can occur (Table 41.2).

Dieting and eating disorders

Many teenage girls experience dissatisfaction with their body image, and attempt to address this by dieting; at any one time, 30% of teenage girls are actively dieting, but the majority will have dieted at some time. Many different diets are followed, and often for relatively short periods of time. All these diets share the common problem of not educating the user into new, healthier eating habits.

More drastic measures, such as use of diuretics, laxatives or self-induced vomiting, may also be employed to lose weight in the short term.

Some teenagers take this chaotic eating behaviour to the extreme, becoming psychologically disturbed. The commonest forms of this are anorexia nervosa and bulimia nervosa (see Chapter 36). Anorexia is up to ten times more common in girls than boys; it is assumed this is due to different pressures related to body image ideals.

Table 41.1 Summary of short- and long-term concerns related to increased prevalence of overweight in children.

Immediate concerns	Long-term concerns
Physical problems reduce ability to participate in peer activities	Likelihood of remaining overweight/obese, increased risk of associated health and social problems
Social isolation, bullying, difficulty in forming peer relationships	Relationship difficulties with partners
Psychological consequences, including low self-esteem, underachievement, mental health problems	Unemployment
Early onset of medical problems, including type 2 diabetes, respiratory problems, sleep apnoea, hypertension, orthopaedic problems	Reduced life expectancy

Table 41.2 Potential risks to nutritional status of children of a poorly constructed vegetarian diet.

Possible threat to nutrition	Possible solution
Lower nutrient density, need to eat larger volumes of food to reach energy needs; problem in children with small appetites	Plan nutrient-rich snacks throughout the day
Avoidance of meat, with no planned substitutes included – risk of low energy and absence of iron, zinc, B vitamins, vitamin D	Ensure meat alternatives included, e.g. pulses, meat replacements based on soya or quorn Include cereal grains and starchy foods to meet energy and nutrient needs
Low intakes of essential fatty acids	Include some green vegetables and seed oils in the diet
Exclusion of dairy products reduces calcium intake	Use calcium-fortified soya products Ensure alternative sources of calcium included
Low-nutrient snacks and soft drinks provide nutrient-poor energy	Avoid these in favour of more nutrient-dense snacks, e.g. dried fruit, nuts

42

Nutrition and early origins of adult disease

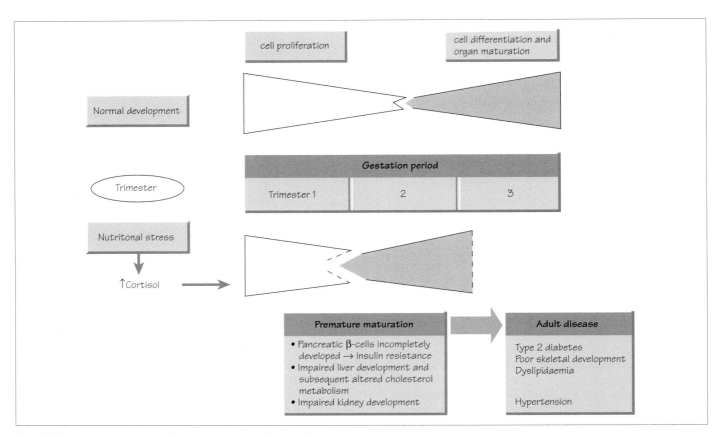

Fig. 42.1 Changes resulting from physiological or nutritional challenges.

Aims

(1) To describe the evidence for a link between fetal development and later risk of disease.

(2) To consider the implications of these findings for maternal nutrition.

An observation that in the UK, rates of coronary heart disease (CHD) in the 1970s followed a similar geographical distribution to infant mortality rates at the beginning of the twentieth century, suggested that influences occurring in infancy may also have a long-term effect on health.

Research has demonstrated a link between the experience of the fetus in the uterine environment, and risk of developing a series of diseases in adult life.

Early evidence

Initial evidence was obtained from birth and early growth records derived from the first decades of the twentieth century in the UK. Records charting neonatal body proportions such as length, head and abdominal circumference and placental weight were also found.

Epidemiologists traced many of these people and recorded their current state of health or, where appropriate, the cause of death.

These early studies showed, across the range of birth weights:

- a statistically significant correlation between lower birth weight and an increased risk of death from cardiovascular disease (CVD);

- in survivors, a higher risk of type 2 diabetes and its markers, and the presence of CVD risk factors (such as hypertension, raised lipid levels and increased levels of blood clotting factors), in those whose birth weight had been lower;

- risk was potentiated by a high adult BMI;

- more recent evidence from many countries has supported these findings, overall showing that for CHD and stroke, there is a 40% difference in risk between the adults who had the highest and lowest birth weights; this persists even when other factors commonly associated with CHD have been taken into account.

Programming

Studies in animal physiology have for many years reported the existence of 'programming' whereby different organs develop at specific stages of gestation. If a physiological insult occurs at this specific time, development will be affected, and the organ or tissue will not be able to recover later.

In addition, cells and tissue exhibit *plasticity*, being able to adapt to particular circumstances. These *adaptations* enable a fetus to survive in adverse conditions. The potential cost of such adaptation, in terms of long-term biological functioning of the individual, is their *potential susceptibility to disease*.

This has been termed the *'thrifty genotype'*, which ensures survival in the womb and continued survival in a deprived environment. However, where the postnatal environment is nutritionally plentiful, these adaptations become a handicap, and may lead to disease.

Developmental consequences

It is recognised that *birth weight* is a very crude measure of fetal development in the womb; a reduced birth weight can arise from slower development of many different tissues. Equally, a normal birth weight may mask disproportionate development of different parts of the body.

Therefore, *variations in body proportions* are believed to indicate different rates of fetal development at different stages of gestation. Different patterns of disproportionate growth have been identified, including:

* shortness (poor overall increase in length);
* thinness (low muscle bulk, low Ponderal Index – weight/height^3);
* large head in relation to trunk (brain growth protected);
* small abdominal circumference (poor organ development);
* disproportionate infant weight in relation to placenta (uneven partitioning of nutrients).

In broad terms it is possible to summarise changes that appear to result from physiological insults or challenges at different stages of pregnancy (Figure 42.1).

(1) Inadequate nutrition at *all stages* of pregnancy results in increased stress either to mother or fetus and results in raised cortisol levels, which affect development of key organs. In particular a series of changes can result in an increased tendency to *hypertension*:
  –maturation of the nephrons in the kidneys is adversely affected;
  –reduced levels of elastin in blood vessels result in stiff arterioles;
  –endothelium-dependent relaxation of blood vessels is impaired due to low levels of nitric oxide production.

(2) In the *second trimester*, poor nutrient supply results in relative insulin resistance and the utilisation of amino acids for energy. This results in poor skeletal muscle development, which persists into post-natal life, and can be linked to later insulin resistance, poor glucose tolerance and the development of *type 2 diabetes*.

(3) In the *third trimester* poor nutrient supplies can result in 'brain sparing', with changes to blood flow diverting nutrients to the brain at the expense of the trunk. This results in poorer development of the liver, and its associated products; consequences include altered ability to control blood cholesterol levels, and blood clotting factors, resulting in increased risk of *dyslipidaemia* and *CHD*.

Links to maternal nutrition

The ability of the mother to provide nutrients to the fetus depends on:
* her own development and ability to sustain good uterine blood flow;
* the quality of the placental development and flow of blood in the umbilical cord;
* the growth of the fetus, which plays a part in regulating its nutrient supply.

All of these can be affected by nutritional status and any constraint will adversely affect fetal growth and development. Evidence supporting this includes:
* *General food shortage* affecting women in a previously well-fed population (Dutch Hunger Winter) has resulted in CHD, obesity, hyperlipidaemias and type 2 diabetes in the offspring, as adults, varying with the stage of pregnancy affected.
* Women with *low BMI*, low weight gain and low triceps skinfolds have offspring with higher blood pressure by adolescence, and increased risk of insulin resistance and dyslipidaemia as adults.
* *Low protein diets* are associated with raised blood pressures in offspring; adding glycine to the diet prevents the rise in blood pressure.
* *Folate* may be a key in early pregnancy diets, by controlling gene expression; ensuring adequate intakes of green vegetables in women on poor diets, increased birth weights.
* *Calcium* supplementation reduces blood pressure in offspring, with no effect on birth weight.

Practical implications

It is important in the light of these findings that girls and young women are nutritionally prepared for pregnancy, so they can fully sustain the nutritional and physiological demands.
* Diets during pregnancy should ensure an adequate supply of all nutrients.
* Babies who are born small should have particular attention paid to them, and they should be targeted for advice to maintain normal body weight and avoid overweight.
* It is the concurrence of a low birth weight, rapid growth in childhood and later overweight in adulthood that imposes the greatest risk of disease.

Possible mechanisms

Many of these mechanisms have been developed from studies in animal models, but they are believed to apply also in humans. However, ethical considerations make such studies in humans difficult.

* During early fetal development cells normally undergo periods of proliferation followed at some later time by cell differentiation. Under normal circumstances this leads to organs being both of the correct size and fully developed.
* The balance between proliferation and differentiation is controlled by cortisol, initially released by the maternal adrenal cortex and towards the later stages of pregnancy augmented by fetal release (mostly after week 23).
* In the early stages of pregnancy maternal cortisol readily passes across the placenta into the fetal circulation.
* Prematurely high levels during this period will lead to organs maturing before they are fully formed (Figure 42.1).
* Maternal undernutrition (particularly low protein and energy intake) represents a physiological stress to the mother, and her response is increased production of cortisol by the adrenal cortex.
* The placenta produces the enzyme 11-β-hydroxysteroid dehydrogenase (HSD), which inactivates cortisol and protects the fetus from excess maternal cortisol levels.
* The enzyme is most effective in the later stages of pregnancy.
* If the mother experiences stress associated with undernutrition in the early months of pregnancy, the fetus is likely to receive abnormally high levels of cortisol, which may interfere with the normal programming of organ development.

43 Nutrition in older adults

Aims

(1) To describe the physiological changes that occur in ageing and their impact on nutrition.

(2) To consider how nutritional vulnerability may be identified and nutritional needs addressed.

Increases in the numbers of people aged over 65, and sharp rises in those aged over 80 and over 90 years, mean that in many Western countries the over-65 age group will soon account for one-quarter of the total population.

The process of ageing

In recent decades it has been noted that the biological changes associated with ageing are occurring later than in the past, so chronological age may be 10 years ahead of biological age. This is believed to be partly attributable to better nutrition and more attention to lifestyle.

Ageing results from the interplay between genetic programming, lifestyle and nutrition; the latter two are within an individual's control, and could be modified to enhance longevity.

Survival mechanisms

Survival is attributable to having good '*maintenance and repair*' *systems* within the body to deal with changes as they occur and limit damage that leads to ageing and disease.

- These systems are *supported by nutrition*, which provides protein, energy and the vitamins and minerals used to maintain homeostasis; most notable are the antioxidant nutrients that limit damage caused by free radicals.
- In parallel, *avoiding factors that cause damage* is also important. For example, toxins such as alcohol, smoking, drugs, excessive intakes of salt, sugar and fat, as well as environmental contaminants like pesticides, additives or preservatives, should be limited as far as possible.

The following help to achieve good nutrition:

- physical activity – this *maintains energy needs* and appetite, ensuring adequate food intake; also maintains muscle mass, which supports independent living and ability to provide oneself with food;
- social interaction – this *encourages eating* and maintains an interest in food;
- selecting food from *a wide variety*, including all food groups in appropriate amounts.

Physiological changes associated with ageing

A number of physiological changes occur with ageing, albeit at different rates and to different extents in individuals (Table 43.1).

Changes linked to **medical conditions** can impact on nutritional status (these may be due to the disease or its treatment):

- reduced mobility – musculoskeletal, neurological, circulatory, respiratory, excess weight;
- cognitive function – impairment and dementia;
- psychological illnesses – including depression (also reactive depression following bereavement), mental illness, alcoholism.

Social factors, including financial status, type of housing, access to shops and facilities, awareness of appropriate meal composition/educational level/cooking skills may also affect food intake.

Assessment of older adults

This group contains a wide age range and a large variation in physical and mental health. Consequently it is difficult to set standards of 'normality' against which individual assessment results can be compared.

It is therefore more effective to adopt a *combination of screening tools*, which include:

- assessment of current health status;
- social and psychological factors;
- food intake and anthropometric measurements;

Table 43.1 Physiological changes associated with ageing and their impact on nutrition.

Physiological change	Potential consequences for nutritional intake
Reduced lean body mass, associated with culturally determined sedentary lifestyle	Lower BMR, smaller energy needs, poorer nutrient intake
Loss of sensory acuity – taste, smell, hearing, vision	Reduced enjoyment of food, inhibits desire for eating
	Less confidence in obtaining and preparing food may limit quantity and variety of food intake
Quality of dentition; dry mouth with reduced saliva flow	Lack of teeth or poorly fitting dentures has detrimental effect on quality and quantity of food intake. Some food groups may be excluded
	Poor oral hygiene causes sores and ulcers, making eating painful
Kidney function reduced	Affects ability to concentrate urine or deal with low fluid intakes
	Risk of dehydration, and subsequent confusional state, including disregarding food intake
Gastrointestinal tract changes, including secretion of hormones, enzymes and acid, reduced motility	Prolonged satiety caused by slow movement along tract, and raised levels of hormones (CCK), reduce appetite
	Reduced acid secretion may affect absorption of minerals from food
	Slow motility may result in constipation, affecting appetite and tendency to use laxatives, which may reduce nutrient absorption
Immune system less efficient, fewer T-lymphocytes produced; may also be stressed by chronic disease states	Adequate nutritional intake of a wide range of nutrients needed to sustain immune system
	Poor immune status increases risk of infection with consequent poor food intake

- haematological measurements;
- biochemical measurements.

Nutritional needs

Because of the diversity in this age group, information about nutritional requirements remains speculative, and is often extrapolated from data based on younger adults.

Energy needs are likely to be lower, due to a reduction in metabolic rate, and reduced physical activity. However, the energy cost of activities, including walking, may be higher than in younger adults.

Protein needs are similar or slightly higher than those of younger adults. Requirements for **minerals** and **vitamins** may also be increased, or be at least the same as in younger adults, due to less efficient absorption and metabolism.

A number of nutrients appear to be less well supplied in the diet of this group and intakes fall below recommended levels (Table 43.2). In addition there is likely to be low biochemical status of these nutrients, with consequent implications for health.

Care for the older adult

A range of care provision for older adults who become nutritionally at risk, includes:

- Community meals – those delivered to people's homes, lunch clubs and sheltered accommodation.
- Residential and nursing homes – provide accommodation and care for the more vulnerable and frail older people, who are more likely to have additional problems, contributing to poorer nutritional status.

Standards and guidelines are in existence to ensure that the provision is appropriate, although studies have indicated that these are not always met.

Table 43.2 Key nutrients that may be at risk in older adults.

Nutrient	Who is at risk of poor intake	Possible health consequences
Energy/protein	Inactive, poor appetite, frail elderly, institutionalised, post-trauma	Poor general nutritional intake – all nutrients low Weight loss, low plasma albumin, poor wound healing, depressed immune status High risk of mortality
B vitamins (including folate, B_6, B_{12}, thiamin and riboflavin)	In cases of atrophic gastritis; heavy drinkers; poor diet, especially low intake of milk, green vegetables	Raised levels of homocysteine, link with cardiovascular disease and Alzheimer's disease Impaired cognitive function Megaloblastic anaemia
Vitamin D	Housebound/institutionalised	Consequences for bone health, immune system and muscle strength Increased risk of bone fracture and loss of independence
Iron	Where there is poor dentition and low meat intake; use of NSAID drugs, causing gastric blood loss. Institutionalised	Poor iron status
Vitamin C	Lower socioeconomic groups; institutionalised	Less resistance to infection, poor wound healing
Potassium	Low fruit and vegetable intakes – associated with poor dentition	Low status, linked with high salt intakes contributes to hypertension. Also poor muscle strength
Zinc	Low food intake, especially little meat	Depressed immune function, increased susceptibility to infection, poor wound healing Reduced taste acuity

44 Nutrition in ethnic minority groups and impact of religion on diet

Aims

(1) To review the dietary practices associated with certain religions.
(2) To consider the potential nutritional implications of these dietary practices.

The nutritional relevance of migration

People may live within countries that are not their own, having migrated there for a number of reasons. There is a long tradition of migration around the world, and the offspring of the original migrants may come to see the host country as their own, or retain a feeling of 'otherness'. One of the key aspects of difference is retention of dietary practices that reflect the 'home' country.

Although these dietary practices may be healthy and balanced, for a variety of reasons they may become less so when practised in the host country, and consequently lead to nutritional vulnerability.

On the other hand it should also be recognised that the dietary practices of many immigrants have enriched the diet of a country's indigenous population, as familiarity with 'ethnic' foods has increased.

Ethnic minority groups in the UK

The 2001 census showed that people belonging to ethnic minority groups represented about 7.9% of the UK population (4.6 million).

This figure also includes people of mixed race, who accounted for 15% of the total.

Influences that may contribute to nutritional risk

- *Discrimination*, which affects many aspects of life – including housing, education, access to shops, access to benefits, and ability to save and invest for the future.
- *Communication difficulties*, affecting access to health care and social integration.
- *Low income*, often linked to poorly paid employment/unemployment – resulting in food poverty.
- *Adaptation of the culturally traditional diet* to include some items from the host country's diet may result in an unbalancing of nutritional intakes, as nutritionally poor snack and convenience items are included.
- Dietary advice on *healthy eating may not be seen as relevant* or appropriate for the dietary customs.
- The balance between 'continuity' and 'change' results in *considerable diversity* for individuals, families and communities, leading to very variable experience and level of risk.

Table 44.1 A summary of the main dietary practices of major religious groups.

Food	Strict Hindus, Sikhs, Jains, Buddhists	Most Hindus	Most Sikhs	Most Muslims	Orthodox Jews	Rastafarians, Seventh Day Adventists
Dietary principle	No killing for food: vegan/vegetarian	May eat some animal food if less strict	May eat some animal food if less strict	Restrictions laid down in Koran; food must be 'halal'	Dietary laws from Bible: permitted food is 'kosher'	Vegetarian diet, believed best for health; fresh food preferred
Beef	No	No	No	Halal	Kosher	No
Pork	No	No	No	No	No	No
Mutton/lamb	No	Probably not	Possibly	Halal	Kosher	No
Chicken	No	Possibly	Possibly	Halal	Kosher	No
Fish	No	Possibly	Possibly	With fins + scales	With fins + scales	Possibly
Milk/yogurt/butter	Yes	Yes	Yes	Yes	Yes	Probably
Cheese	Homemade	Vegetarian	Possibly	Possibly	Vegetarian	Possibly
Eggs	No	Probably	Possibly	Yes	Yes	Possibly
Oils/fats	Vegetable oil/ghee	Ghee/groundnut/mustard oil	Vegetable oil/ghee	Groundnut oil/vegetable oil	Kosher margarine/vegetable oil	Vegetable oil
Alcohol	No	Probably not	Probably not	No	Kosher wine for ritual use	No
Fasting	Yes: individual and at festivals	Yes: individual and at festivals	Yes: individual, mainly women	Yes: prescribed	Yes: prescribed, linked to festivals	Yes: individual
Other aspects	Humoral theory of health important, balanced with foods	Hot/cold (humoral) theory of health applied	Fewer restrictions	May avoid processed foods for fear of forbidden ingredients	Milk and meat intake separated by 3–6 hours. Separated in food preparation	May avoid additives, seasonings and condiments

The main groups are:
- Europeans (from all member states of the European Union (EU) and other European countries);
- Asians from the Indian subcontinent – Indian, Pakistani and Bangladeshi people (account for half of the total);
- Black Caribbean and Black African (account for one-quarter of the total);
- Chinese, from Singapore, Hong Kong, Vietnam and China.

In addition, there are people from all parts of the world, but their diets are either:
- relatively well integrated into those of the British population (possibly sharing many of the dietary problems); or
- insufficiently studied because the groups are too small or widely dispersed.

Religion and diet
Religious adherence has an important influence on dietary practices for many people in these groups (Table 44.1).

Dietary restriction is reported to be practised by 80–95% of the groups of Asian origin. The main religious groups are Muslim, Hindu and Sikh. Other religious groups among whom diets are likely to be altered include Jews, Buddhists, Rastafarians and Seventh Day Adventists.

Adherence to religious practice is important as part of a sense of faith and belonging, but will nevertheless *vary in its rigidity* between individuals.

Nutritional issues
In the UK, most nutritional issues have been studied in the two largest ethnic minority groups, Asians (from the Indian subcontinent) and Black Caribbean and African people. These include:

(1) *Infant birth weight*: lower birth weights, especially in Pakistani mothers, linked to poorer iron and vitamin D status. This continues into second generation births.

(2) *Infant feeding*: colostrum may be withheld, having implications for transfer of immunity to baby. Also later weaning, and high levels of cow's milk use recorded, with implications for infant's iron status. It is important to ensure good advice on use of a mixed weaning diet with iron-containing foods.

(3) *Eating away from home*: some may eat 'Western' style food away from home, provided it complies with restrictions. Foods from 'takeaways' and sandwiches may be bought. In institutions (e.g. hospital) food provision may not appeal, even when it is 'acceptable' according to dietary laws. This may have implications for the implementation of dietetic treatment.

(4) *Nutritional anaemias*: iron deficiency is recorded in 25–30% of women in Asian and Black Caribbean groups, approximately three times higher than in the general population. These ethnic differences are not seen in men. Children also exhibit twice the level of iron deficiency anaemia than that in White counterparts. Folate deficiency resulting in anaemia is reported in women, especially in pregnancy; rates are three times greater than in White control groups.

Folate intakes tend to be low because of cooking methods used, with prolonged heating of potential sources.

(5) *Vitamin D deficiency*: still occurs despite campaigns to raise awareness of the need for vigilance on vitamin D. Low plasma levels of vitamin D found across all members of households, suggesting a predominantly dietary origin, linked to degrees of vegetarianism (diets containing little vitamin D and calcium). Most common in Hindu families, particularly affects women of childbearing age and older women.

(6) *Nutrition-related non-communicable diseases (NR-NCDs)*: central obesity is more prevalent than in the general population in both the Asian and African minority groups. Associated with this is a higher prevalence of type 2 diabetes (in both men and women) and coronary heart disease (particularly in men), both of which are two to three times greater than in the White population, and develop at a younger age. The African Caribbean population carries a higher risk of stroke rather than coronary heart disease.

Awareness of risk and acceptance of the need to change is often difficult to communicate, so the diseases are identified late, often when complications have already developed.

Health promotion needs to provide accurate information and make change an easy option for these communities, by attempting to remove barriers.
- These may include a reluctance to take up physical activity, especially by women, who may be restricted in their movement outside the home. Leisure centres and swimming pools have a role to play in organising 'women only' sessions.
- Introducing healthier cooking methods, while promoting the beneficial aspects of traditional diets, requires sympathetic and informed intervention.
- One of the tools used in education about the diet is the Balance of Good Health (see Chapter 8). Variants of the original UK diet-based model have been developed to identify foods that are traditional to different diets. These can be used with the appropriate communities to demonstrate relevance of the guidelines to their own diets.
- Successful schemes have trained members of the communities to act as advocates for change, while at the same time promoting greater integration and reducing isolation.

Risk factors for NR-NCDs
Studies of the causes and risk factors for NR-NCDs in these groups have identified a number of possible indicators, including:
- high incidence of smoking and poverty-affected lifestyle (especially Bangladeshi and Pakistani groups);
- higher risk of raised blood pressure (high salt intake in African Caribbean group);
- short stature, increases risk;
- higher levels of lipoprotein(a) in Asian men;
- small babies, rapid weight gain in early life;
- low folate status, raises homocysteine levels;
- low levels of physical activity (not a cultural norm).

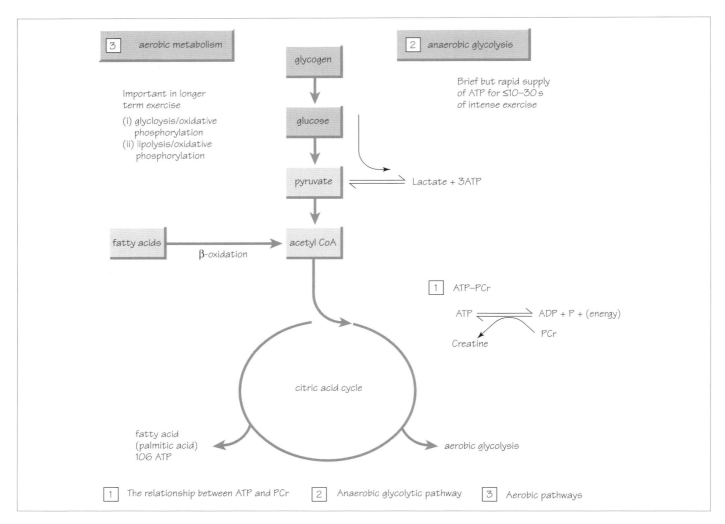

Fig. 45.1 Energy substrates and metabolic pathways: ATP production from different substrates (per mol).

Aims

(1) To consider how energy is used in physical exercise and major determinants of sources of energy.

Increased physical activity requires energy to be supplied at an increased rate to active muscles. Although the energy requirement of a sedentary adult is approximately 7.5–11.5 MJ (1800–2800 kcal)/day this can increase to as much as 36 MJ (9000 kcal)/day for extreme endurance events (e.g. cyclists competing in the mountain section of the 'Tour de France'). However, the energy needs of the majority of athletes will be more moderate, around 14.5–18 MJ (3500–4500 kcal)/day, depending on the sport and level of training.

Adenosine triphosphate (ATP)

ATP is the fundamental molecule that on breakdown to ADP provides energy for contracting muscle. ATP stores are very limited and require continual replenishment; the amount stored would fuel only about two seconds of exercise. The main routes for maintaining ATP stores are shown in Figures 45.1 and 45.2.

Energy supply

Carbohydrates (in the form of glycogen and glucose) and fats (fatty acids) are the two main sources of energy. Protein makes a small (10–15%) contribution to total energy expenditure, generally towards the end of a period of endurance exercise.

An important principle is that carbohydrates are the preferred energy source particularly for more intense and prolonged exercise. To understand why different energy substrates are used under different circumstances a brief review of the relevant metabolic pathways is required.

Importance of lipids as substrate

• CHO stores in muscle (300–800 g) and liver (80 g) are limited; fats stored mainly in subcutaneous tissue are found in very much *greater amounts* (minimum 5 kg in males, more in females).

• Lipids are considerably more *energy dense* than CHOs. Metabolism of one gram of fat will deliver considerably more ATP molecules

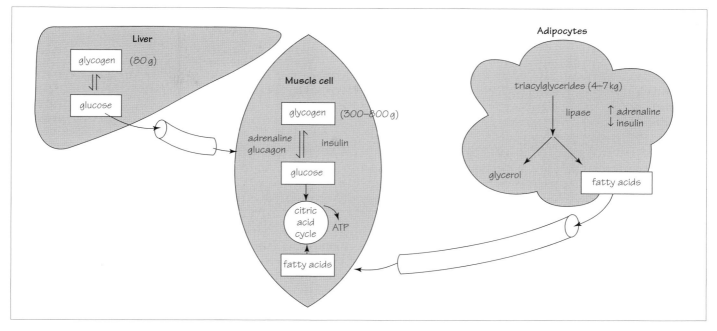

Fig. 45.2 Location of major energy substrates and the main endocrine control factors.

than one gram of CHO; however, more oxygen is required to metabolise fats, and fats cannot be metabolised anaerobically (Figure 45.2).

Factors determining substrate use

The proportions of ATP derived from CHO and fat depend upon a number of factors:

Duration and intensity of exercise (see Table 45.1)

Key issues in maximising energy supply are:
• Glycogen levels – are crucial in enabling high-intensity exercise to be continued.
• Even relatively small amounts of energy from lipid breakdown during high-intensity exercise help to protect muscle glycogen stores and increase the time to exhaustion when stores are depleted.
• Maintaining blood glucose levels is essential, as a reduction will

impair accuracy and judgement in performance, and contribute to fatigue. Dietary intervention to support blood glucose is essential.
• Levels of insulin, adrenaline and glucagon are important in determining which substrates are used in different circumstances.

Level of training

Training increases aerobic fitness. This has several benefits:
• increase in blood supply to muscle, thus enabling faster delivery of oxygen;
• increase in levels of enzymes for aerobic metabolism;
• more rapid establishment of fat metabolism as energy substrate, and therefore better protection of CHO reserves.

Diet

The nature of an athlete's diet will significantly affect her or his ability to train and perform. This is discussed in Chapter 46.

Table 45.1 Summary of the effects of duration and intensity of exercise on substrate use.

Level of exercise	Main substrate for muscle contraction	Comments
At rest/minimal physical exercise	Lipid metabolism	CNS and RBCs require glucose for metabolism
Brief intense exercise (up to 10s)	Anaerobic breakdown of ATP and PCr	In muscle, PCr is found in concentrations about four times that of ATP, used to recreate ATP during brief rest periods
Intense exercise (up to 90s)	Anaerobic metabolism of glucose or glycogen to pyruvate, with net formation of two or three ATP units respectively	Lactate later has to be reconverted to glucose. Useful for short sprints before physiological adjustments have occurred
Medium-term intense exercise	Partly by anaerobic breakdown of glycogen or glucose, increasingly by aerobic metabolism	This yields more energy to sustain exercise
Light to moderate exercise	Lipid metabolism makes an increasingly significant contribution and CHO correspondingly less	Related to changes in hormone levels; adrenaline secretion stimulates lipolysis, and insulin is inhibited; may take 20 minutes to reach a steady state
Moderately high levels of sustained exercise	Lipids are the main energy substrate. Depleted muscle glycogen eventually results in fatigue and terminates the exercise	Muscle glycogen stores are reduced and gluconeogenesis in the liver (predominantly from glycerol from fat breakdown or later amino acid residues from protein) becomes important to maintain blood glucose levels

46 Nutrition and sport II

Aims

(1) To identify nutritional requirements for exercise and how these can be met.

(2) To consider some dietary supplements used in sport.

The diet consumed by an athlete is a critical element of the athlete's training and performance (Table 46.1). Nutritional goals will vary depending on the sport, and may aim for endurance, speed or power/strength. In addition, actual body mass may be important, especially in aesthetic sports (such as gymnastics) or where there are specific weight categories for competition (rowers, combat sports, jockeys). Large body mass may also be desirable in other sports, such as weight lifting and body building.

Importance of carbohydrate in the general diet

A common feature of the dietary advice offered to athletes either in training or in competition is the need to increase or maintain carbohydrate stores.

Time to exhaustion or duration of maximal effort can be increased by ensuring that glycogen stores are maximally filled with glycogen. This can be achieved by ensuring an adequate CHO intake (7–10 g/kg body weight per day). This is important for:

> ### CHO loading
>
> Supercompensation of muscle glycogen stores can be achieved by a technique known as CHO loading. This is relevant where duration of exercise exceeds 90–120 minutes; time to exhaustion can be increased by 20%.
>
> The technique involves a high CHO intake with tapered exercise and rest for 3–4 days prior to competition. A potential drawback of such supercompensation is that glycogen is stored with water (2.7 g/g glycogen). This can make the muscles feel heavy, and requires the athlete to become accustomed to the sensation.

- maintaining sufficient energy supplies for regular training;
- preparing for a competition/event.

In the latter case, 24–36 hours of rest with an adequate CHO intake will ensure that glycogen stores are replete.

Carbohydrate before exercise

Topping up glycogen stores is important in the last hours before exercise. A pre-exercise meal, rich in CHO of low and medium GI (200–300 g), will ensure a steady release of CHO over several hours. The meal should preferably be low in fat and fibre to allow for easy digestion and have a low to moderate protein content.

In the last hour before exercise, high-GI CHO may be taken, although in a few athletes this may lead to release of insulin and inhibition of lipolysis in early exercise. Testing the effects of pre-exercise CHO ingestion is advised to gauge individual response.

Carbohydrate during exercise

Consuming CHO drinks during an event lasting more than 45 minutes is important. This serves the following purposes:

- maintains blood glucose levels and brain function;
- provides additional fluid to prevent dehydration;
- delays the onset of fatigue.

A CHO intake of approximately 60 g/h is recommended. The majority of CHO-containing drinks are isotonic (4–8 g CHO per 100 mL), providing a readily absorbable source of CHO, and electrolytes that facilitate the absorption.

Absorption is also faster if there is already fluid in the stomach, hence athletes are advised to start exercise with at least 300–500 mL fluid in the stomach.

Carbohydrate after exercise

After exercise, muscles need to be refuelled as rapidly as possible with glycogen to allow more exercise to be undertaken later, or on subsequent days.

Table 46.1 Summary of dietary principles in exercise and sport.

Nutrient	Advice	Reasons/benefits
Carbohydrate	Maintain intakes up to 7–10 g/kg during training and competition. Attention to intake prior to, during and after exercise	Keeps muscle glycogen levels topped up, and allows maximal performance. Before exercise – tops up glycogen stores. During exercise – protects blood glucose levels, delays fatigue. After exercise – allows rapid replenishment of glycogen stores
Protein	Most athletes already consume sufficient protein in a mixed diet. May need attention in vegetarian athletes, or where food and energy intakes are very low (e.g. in low body weight sports)	Needed for muscle maintenance and repair. Also to maintain immune function
Fat	May need to include average amounts of fat (35% of energy) in the diet if energy needs are high	Type of fat eaten should follow healthy eating advice. Fat-soluble vitamin intakes may be compromised by very low-fat diets
Minerals and vitamins	Balanced diet provides adequate levels. Athletes with low overall dietary intakes may need supplements. Attention particularly to antioxidant nutrients	Female athletes may need additional iron if intakes low. Low body weight athletes risk low calcium status and may need to take additional calcium
Fluid	Essential to maintain hydration; habitual intake important	Fluid with electrolytes and CHO is useful to provide efficient absorption and maintain CHO levels

Glycogen synthesis in muscles is enhanced in the 2 hours after exercise; taking advantage of this allows more glycogen to be stored. An intake of CHO of 1–2 g/kg body weight is suggested.

Refuelling diets should therefore contain high-GI CHO initially, perhaps as snacks or drinks, followed by a meal of low- and medium-GI CHO to sustain the supply of glucose to the muscles over a period of time. Including protein in the meal enhances glycogen storage and may also benefit immune function, which can be compromised after exercise.

Protein needs in exercise

Protein does not contribute significantly to the energy supply in exercise. However, there is potentially an increase in protein requirement because:

- muscle fibrils are damaged in exercising muscles leading to an increased need for protein for repair;
- when athletes first start to train, the exercise causes hypertrophy of muscles, which increases protein needs to achieve a positive nitrogen balance.

Recommended protein intakes are therefore 1.2–1.7 g/kg body weight, depending on the sport. In practice, this level of protein is typically consumed in the normal Western diet. Additional focus on protein or protein supplements is therefore not needed to reach these intakes.

There is no evidence of any advantage of intakes above 2 g/kg, and a possible danger that this amount of protein in the diet will compromise the amount of CHO eaten, and limit the ability to exercise.

Dietary supplements and sport

With the exception of energy intake the evidence that normal dietary supplements enhance sporting performance is poor. Although free radical production increases during exercise there is little evidence that vitamin C or E supplementation protects against oxidative damage. A very large number of ergogenic aids are marketed and used by athletes; however, for the vast majority there is no clear evidence of improved performance.

Creatine

Creatine plays an important part in energy delivery to muscles (see Figure 45.1). In the early 1990s the oral intake of creatine (2–3 g/day) became popular. Supplementary creatine:

- significantly increases muscle creatine levels;
- may delay the onset of fatigue; and
- may improve high-intensity work levels.

Intermittent, short but intensive bouts of exercise appear to be improved most and endurance events to benefit least.

Caffeine

Ingested an hour before exercise, caffeine:

- increases plasma fatty acid levels;
- increases recruitment of muscle fibres;
- has beneficial effects on cognitive function (primarily psychomotor skill and attention).

Even low doses of caffeine (5 mg/kg body weight) increase time to exhaustion when working at very high levels of activity. The International Olympic Committee allows a maximum of 12 mg/mL urine.

47 Adverse reactions to food I

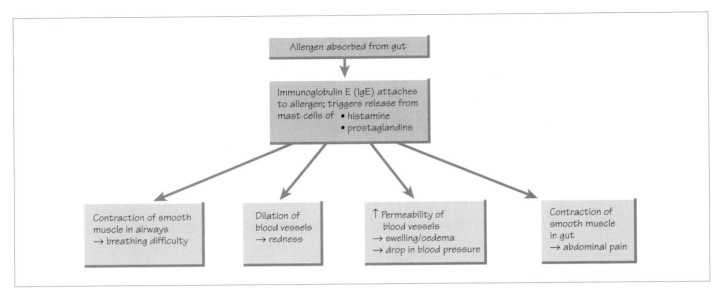

Allergen absorbed from gut

↓

Immunoglobulin E (IgE) attaches to allergen; triggers release from mast cells of • histamine • prostaglandins

Contraction of smooth muscle in airways → breathing difficulty

Dilation of blood vessels → redness

↑ Permeability of blood vessels → swelling/oedema → drop in blood pressure

Contraction of smooth muscle in gut → abdominal pain

Fig. 47.1 Possible consequences in an IgE-mediated allergic reaction.

Aims

(1) To introduce the range of possible adverse reactions to food.
(2) To consider allergic reactions to food.

It has been reported that up to one in three people may suffer an allergic reaction at some time in their lives. Only a proportion of these, however, are triggered by food.

There are a number of adverse reactions to food, including:
- food intolerance, which includes allergic reactions;
- food poisoning;
- food aversion.

Food intolerance

Food intolerance is a generic name covering a range of responses to a specific food or nutrient that are *reproducible*. Food intolerance includes:
- allergic reactions (which may be immunoglobulin E (IgE) mediated, or non- IgE mediated);
- pharmacological reactions;
- enzyme reactions.

Allergic reactions: IgE-mediated reactions

Allergic responses (usually to proteins in foods) are mediated by the immune system.

The reactions involve immunoglobulins, which trigger mast cells to release histamine and prostaglandins. The cascade of events is shown in Figure 47.1. It can involve a number of systems of the body, including:
- respiratory system;
- the skin;
- blood vessels;
- gastrointestinal tract;
- nervous system.

Prevalence of food intolerance

Attempting to record the prevalence of food intolerance is notoriously difficult partly because of differences in definitions and also in methodologies. For example:
- questionnaires may introduce bias;
- diagnosis using challenge tests is time consuming;
- tests are often not very sensitive;
- the range of potentially allergenic foodstuffs is enormous;
- the time course of a response may be immediate or delayed, making it difficult to attribute to a specific allergen.

A study in the UK found that in a sample of 18 000 people, 20% reported food intolerance. However, following controlled challenges it was found that only 1–2% of the adult population exhibit food intolerance, and for children the figure was 5–8%.

The severity of the reaction varies between individuals, and may be localised to a single site. However, if a reaction affects a number of systems, there may be a generalised fall in blood pressure, resulting in anaphylactic shock, and the need for immediate medical attention. Individuals who are aware of their risks are generally advised to carry adrenaline to counter this reaction.

The increasing prevalence of *peanut allergies* in young children is probably linked to the early introduction of peanut proteins found in peanut butter, cereals, confectionery and baked goods. Such children are extremely sensitive to peanut proteins and even 100 µg can provoke an anaphylactic response. Complete avoidance of peanuts and their derivatives (and other nuts and pulses) is vital.

Most adults do not develop allergies in later life, the only major exception being shellfish allergy.

Development of an allergic reaction

- Most potential allergens derived from the diet do not trigger responses because of the presence of secretory immunoglobulin A (IgA) lining the gut.
- However, this protection is absent during the first few months of life and allergic reactions are more commonly established in this period.
- Breast milk contains IgA and may confer some protection.
- In children, cow's milk, eggs, soya beans and soya products, fish, wheat, tree nuts, vegetables and fruit are most likely to trigger early allergies.
- Although children generally grow out of most food allergies, those to peanuts, tree nuts, fish and shellfish may be retained. Children who develop IgE-mediated reactions to milk or eggs often exhibit allergic responses in later life to house dust and pollen.

Possible explanations for increased prevalence of allergies

Although genetic predisposition has a significant part to play in determining vulnerability to allergic disease it cannot explain the increase in the prevalence of allergic responses observed in children over recent years.

A number of explanations may account for this:

- Low birth-weight babies (for gestational age) are more likely to develop allergies in the first year of life. Disrupted fetal development may account for this phenomenon.
- Children are exposed to fewer infectious diseases because of a greater awareness of the need for hygiene; consequently the immune system may be less well developed. The immune response then becomes exaggerated when challenged with harmless antigens.
- Breastfeeding only occurs in a proportion of infants, depriving some infants of immunological protection.
- Contemporary diets contain a higher proportion of n-6 fatty acids, which are associated with more pro-inflammatory eicosanoids, including prostaglandins, which have important roles in allergic responses. Intakes of n-3 fatty acids, which could counterbalance this effect, are relatively low.
- The early introduction of allergenic substances into the infant diet, at a time when the gut is immature and able to absorb whole antigens. Use of wheat-based cereals and soya products may be particularly harmful at this stage. Use of baby rice, potatoes, fruit and vegetables is recommended for early weaning.

The Food Standards Agency has recently published a list of food constituents that must be identified on food labels, and that represent the most commonly occurring allergens in the UK diet. This is shown in Table 47.2.

Non-IgE-mediated reactions, other types of food intolerance and adverse reactions to food are considered in Chapter 48.

Table 47.2 List of food constituents that must be identified on food labels in the UK, as representing potential allergens.

Cereals containing gluten:	Crustaceans	*Nuts:*
Wheat	Eggs	Almonds
Rye	Fish	Hazelnuts
Barley	Peanuts	Walnuts
Oats	Soya beans	Cashew
Spelt	Milk	Pecan
Kamut	Celery	Brazil
Hybridised strains	Mustard	Pistachio
	Sesame seed	Macadamia
	Sulphur dioxide and sulphites	Queensland nuts

Aims

(1) To consider food intolerances other than those that are IgE mediated.
(2) To consider food poisoning and food aversion, as adverse reactions to food.
(3) To introduce means of diagnosis for adverse reactions.

Food intolerances

Non-IgE-mediated reactions to food

Not all adverse reactions to food involve IgE- and histamine-mediated events, as described in Chapter 47. Other elements of the immune system, including T-lymphocytes and scavenger cells, may become involved in reactions, which may take several hours or days to develop fully.

The most common example of a non-IgE-mediated reaction is *coeliac disease*, in which genetically susceptible people respond to gluten found in wheat, barley, rye and some varieties of oats.

In addition a number of other non-IgE-mediated allergic conditions have been investigated but not necessarily confirmed:

- Urticaria and dermatitis
- Infant colic
- Irritable bowel syndrome
- Asthma
- Migraine
- Attention deficit hyperactivity disorder (ADHD)
- Rheumatoid arthritis

Attempting to identify foods that trigger symptoms in these conditions is often a difficult task. There is often inconsistency of findings between subjects for trigger foods, so individual advice may be needed.

There is a danger that a wide range of foods is apparently found to trigger symptoms, and these are excluded from the diet. Consequently there is a risk of nutritional deficiency, if careful dietary planning is not undertaken at the same time.

Coeliac disease

In patients with coeliac disease, dietary gluten leads to reductions in the number and complexity of villi lining the lumen of the gut, primarily in the small intestine. The resulting reduction in surface area for absorption leads to malabsorption of nutrients. The skin may also be affected with an itchy blistering rash on the knees, thighs and elbows.

The condition may remain undiagnosed for a number of years in adults when folate and iron deficiencies lead to anaemia, or inadequate calcium and vitamin D absorption results in poor bone development, or osteoporosis.

Traditionally coeliac disease was confirmed following small bowel biopsy; however, more recently serological tests for antibodies in blood have been developed.

Pharmacological reactions

Some foods contain pharmacological agents that may cause allergic reactions. However, the amounts needed are much greater than for the allergic reactions discussed above. Examples include:

- cheeses (Roquefort, Parmesan and mature Cheddar);
- wine (and other fermented products);
- bananas, yeast extract, avocados, chocolate, oranges and some fish products, which can contain biogenic amines such as histamine, tyramine, phenylethylamine and octopamine (depending on the food);
- chocolate, tomatoes and strawberries can directly cause release of histamine;
- caffeine can also trigger a pharmacological reaction in sensitive individuals.

Enzyme defects

These may be responsible for food intolerances, causing unpleasant symptoms in certain people. Examples include:

- *Congenital lactase deficiency:* is rare although the enzyme may disappear after infancy and compromise the digestion of milk and milk products. Other disaccharide enzyme activities may be affected by drug therapies or binge or chronic alcohol consumption. In these circumstances symptoms of intolerance occur, including bloating and diarrhoea, as a result of the bacterial fermentation of lactose.

Table 48.1 Summary of different forms of food poisoning.

Causative agent	Symptoms	Vector/food type/agent
Toxins in foods	Diarrhoea and\or vomiting often within minutes of consuming the food Neurotoxins produce muscle paralysis and disruption of nerve transmission Kidney and liver damage	Undercooked red kidney beans Puffer fish (tetrodotoxin) Cereal fungi (ergot) Peanuts (aflatoxin)
Bacteria	Diarrhoea and vomiting, usually within a few hours Some cases of food poisoning may cause serious damage to liver, kidneys or nervous system, and may be fatal in the young or old	*Campylobacter* – most common form of bacterial gastroenteritis in the UK (poultry, meat) *Salmonella* (eggs and poultry) *Escherichia coli* (cold meats)
Bacteria releasing toxins		*Staphylococcus aureus* *Bacillus cereus* *Clostridium botulinum* Found in: eggs, poultry, cold meats, rice and spices
Viruses (most commonly small round structured viruses, SRSV)	Gastroenteritis	Shellfish, but spread by food handlers; can pass rapidly through closed communities, such as hospitals, hotels, schools. Very infectious

- Genetically determined absence of alcohol dehydrogenase in some populations results in the inability to metabolise alcohol.
- Fructose intolerance results in incomplete fructose metabolism, which leads to hypoglycaemia.

There are also a number of other genetically determined enzyme defects, principally affecting amino acid metabolism, that require lifelong dietary modifications.

Food poisoning

Food poisoning is defined as any disease of an infectious or toxic nature associated with contaminated food or water. Table 48.1 summarises the different forms of food poisoning. Good hygiene practices in food production and storage, both on a large scale and in the home, can reduce the risk of these cases.

Food aversion

This relates to unpleasant reactions to food that are not reproduced when the food is covertly presented. Many children are reluctant to eat some vegetables because they regard the taste as being unpleasant.

In some cases people believe there is a link between a food eaten and previous episodes of sickness or gastrointestinal upset. An aversion then develops, which is a learned response and is not associated with a pathological response to a nutrient. These responses, which may be very significant (e.g hyperventilation), are said to be of psychosomatic origin. Interestingly, studies have shown that in many patients such reactions are reduced following psychotherapeutic treatment. They may be of little nutritional significance in most subjects, unless the aversion extends to many foods, or ones that are important sources of nutrients.

Diagnosing adverse reactions to foods

Rigorous testing using strict criteria must be adopted before the existence of an adverse reaction to a food can be confirmed. This will involve:
- excluding the food from the diet and noting that the symptoms disappear and that they reappear when the food is reintroduced;
- taking great care if there is any suspicion of anaphylaxis; such testing must be done under clinical supervision;
- taking a detailed history of diet and symptoms to identify possible triggers; testing of foods must be done using the double-blind technique, when neither the subject nor the tester knows when the food is being introduced.

Tests for allergy include:
- the skin prick test;
- assay of IgE levels;
- intestinal biopsy or intestinal permeability may be carried out in the clinical setting.

Many tests are commercially available to the public. Most have not been adequately validated and are not considered to be reliable in the diagnosis of food allergy.

They may actually represent a danger to the public in that they may result in misdiagnosis and the introduction of harmful exclusion diets, which in the case of children may be particularly hazardous. Dietary changes should ideally only be introduced under the supervision of a dietitian.

There is recognition that services for sufferers from allergies are poor in the UK, and often lack coordination. Proposals have been made for a reorganisation of these services and more training offered to produce a larger number of properly qualified practitioners.

49 Overweight and obesity: aetiological factors

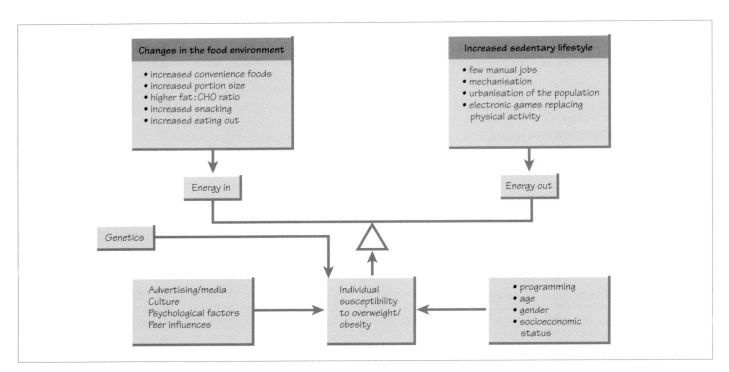

Fig. 49.1 An overview of factors that contribute to changes in energy balance.

Aims
(1) To define overweight and obesity and consider their prevalence.
(2) To consider the contributory factors in energy intake and energy output that lead to overweight and obesity.

Definition
Overweight and obesity can be defined as an excessive accumulation of body fat. In men, a healthy level of body fat may be 15% of total weight; in women this may be 25%, reflecting the hormonal differences and needs between the sexes.

Excessive accumulations of fat may exceed 50% of total weight, contributing to major pathological consequences.

Measuring body fat is not a straightforward process. Several simple surrogate measurements are used to categorise overweight and obesity. These are:
- body mass index;
- waist circumference;
- waist:hip ratio.

See Chapter 3 for further details.

Prevalence of overweight and obesity
Global prevalence has been rising steeply over the last 20 years in most countries; there are now more overweight than undernourished people across the globe.
- Overweight and obesity combined now affects 65% of men and 56% of women in the UK. The figures represent a doubling of prevalence in women and a tripling in men since 1980.

- Obesity affects 22% of men and 23% of women in the UK.
- Rates of overweight and obesity are increasing among children and adolescents.
- In general obesity increases with age.
- Obesity is more prevalent in lower socioeconomic groups in Western countries. However, in some parts of the world, such as India, it is seen more commonly among the more affluent groups.

Public health concerns regarding these trends relate to the parallel increase in risk of associated diseases.
- Obesity is directly responsible for some 6% of all deaths in the Western world and reduces life expectancy by an average of 9 years.
- It is associated with substantial morbidity, in terms of physical, metabolic and psychological consequences.
- The associated financial costs of obesity are estimated to account for 2–8% of health-care budgets in the West, and after diabetes, constitute the second greatest area of expenditure in these budgets.

External influences on energy intake
Food availability
Both the quantity and the nature of the food available to people in many parts of the world has changed substantially in the last decades. Changes include:
- greater choice, with more variety encouraging intake;
- food on sale around the clock;
- improved preservation methods, so food can be always available;
- many foods require little preparation, so can be eaten immediately.

Development of overweight and obesity

Weight gain occurs when the energy intake exceeds the energy output over a period of time.

This represents a *positive energy balance*, such that the energy supplied to the body as food is not used and is therefore stored in adipose tissue.

A reduction in energy intake, an increase in energy output, or both, are needed to remove the stored energy, create *a negative energy balance* and reduce body weight.

Control of energy balance

Physiological control mechanisms exist, to regulate both energy intake and output. These are discussed further in Chapter 21.

For humans in modern society, both intake and output are subject to a variety of external influences. These interact with or override the internal regulatory mechanisms, creating a challenge to the maintenance of energy balance. In addition, the relative importance of these influences varies, as a result of the underlying genetic make-up of the individual, dietary complexity and environmental variables.

Food quantity and quality

Dietary surveys suggest that energy intakes in the UK have fallen since the 1970s. Recorded intakes are frequently under-reported, which makes comparisons with energy output difficult. Nevertheless, the rising incidence of obesity implies that energy intakes still exceed expenditure.

Changes that play a part include:
• increased consumption of convenience, ready prepared or 'fast' food, which has a higher energy density than typical traditional diets, resulting in 'passive overconsumption' of energy;
• a trend to larger portion sizes becoming the norm, which also inadvertently increases food intake;
• people eating a rising proportion of their meals away from home, hence the impact of the food industry on food quality and quantity becomes more pertinent to obesity trends.

Snacking and 'grazing'

A trend away from eating regular meals, to a less structured food intake, typified by consumption of snack and convenience foods and soft drinks throughout the day, rather than eating to satiety at greater intervals. Such intakes tend to be high in fat and high-glycaemic carbohydrate, as well as being generally poor sources of slowly absorbable carbohydrate and micronutrients. The body's appetite control mechanisms are undermined in this way.

Psychological aspects

Attitudes and beliefs have a major impact on food intake. For any one individual, food intake could be affected by:
• their mood and mental state;
• personality;
• self-image and culturally determined body images;
• socialised attitude to food;
• external factors such as peer effects, advertising and media influences.

External influences on energy output

Increased mechanisation

Technological advances result in less need to use human muscle power to carry out energy-demanding manual tasks.
• There are now fewer occupations that can be classified as heavy manual work, and even tasks that were not very physically demanding have been lightened with robots and computer-driven technology. Fewer have physically demanding jobs in agriculture, as urbanisation proceeds rapidly.
• Transport has become increasingly concentrated on the use of the car, as opposed to walking and use of bicycles.

Leisure activity

Secular trends suggest reduced participation in active leisure pursuits.
• The widespread availability of computers and electronic home entertainment systems reduces outdoor leisure activities.
• Physical activity has for many become an item to schedule into the day, with a trip to the gym or swimming pool, rather than an intrinsic part of existence, as it was in the past.
• Increased urbanisation and road traffic, together with safety fears, make outdoor activity less pleasant and compound the problem.

Individual susceptibility

Not everyone exposed to the same external influences on intake or output will experience weight gain. There is a heritable element, although this remains difficult to quantify and separate from environmental influences within families.

Genetics

In some inherited conditions there is a clear link with obesity; most notable among these are Prader–Willi and Bardet–Biedel syndromes.

For the great majority of cases of obesity, the rapid increase in the incidence within a genetically stable population indicates that external factors play the major role. This does not exclude a genetic origin to susceptibility to obesity, which becomes expressed as a result of external changes.

Ethnicity

There are observed differences in patterns of weight gain between different ethnic groups, including body fat distribution and levels of adiposity at particular BMI values.

Vulnerable periods

Research from a number of areas suggests that there are periods during the life cycle when susceptibility to obesity may be programmed (in the fetus and infant) or be increased (during periods of rapid growth, including pregnancy and lactation). The latter may be linked to changes in levels of specific hormones. Age and gender are compounding factors, with patterns of weight gain in adult life differing between men and women.

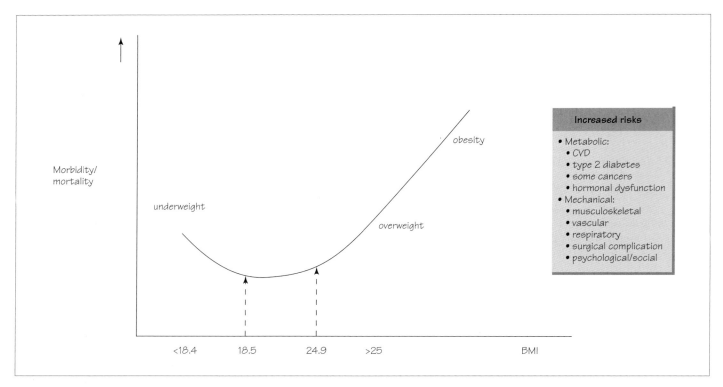

Fig. 50.1 Relationship between BMI and risk of morbidity and mortality.

Aims

(1) To identify some of the major health consequences associated with obesity.

(2) To describe the association between obesity and CVD.

There is a well-recognised relationship between the prevalence of overweight and obesity and rates of morbidity and mortality worldwide. Health risks are related to BMI in a J-shaped relationship (Figure 50.1).

(At the lower end of the BMI range – usually below 19 – risk increases due to the possibility of concurrent illness that causes loss of weight, such as cancer or complications of malnutrition.)

Above a BMI of 25, and especially above 30, there is a progressive increase in morbidity and mortality, associated with a range of factors; these are summarised in Table 50.1.

The metabolic effects in particular are associated with an increased waist circumference; these are likely to result in increased mortality. The remaining effects contribute to morbidity, but eventually indirectly to mortality.

The metabolic effects associated with insulin abnormalities are discussed in Chapter 51.

Cardiovascular disease (CVD)

Obesity is a major risk factor for CVD, and data consistently show a higher incidence of disease with increasing BMI. However, obesity is also a risk factor in a number of the other conditions associated with CVD, such as dyslipidaemia, type 2 diabetes mellitus (and insulin resistance) and hypertension. It is therefore very difficult to separate the attributable risk to each of these comorbidities, as in addition, their relative contributions may differ between individuals.

Overall, it is estimated that in subjects exhibiting the full spectrum of these conditions, CVD mortality is increased threefold; 18% of the variance in CVD risk has been attributed to insulin resistance. It is clear that the deposition of large amounts of fat within the body alters normal metabolic functions and results in a number of potentially harmful changes.

Hypertension

There are several proposed mechanisms that offer an explanation for the high correlation between obesity and hypertension. These include:

• Increase in blood volume as a result of greater salt retention; this is attributed to an antinatriuretic effect of raised insulin levels.

• Changes in hormone levels affect blood pressure regulation; e.g. cortisol production by adipose tissue increases, leptin and angiotensinogen released from adipose tissue have direct hypertensive effects.

• Higher salt intakes and low levels of physical fitness may contribute.

Obesity and cancer

Prevention of overweight is considered to be one of the strategies to

Table 50.1 Pathological consequences of overweight and obesity.

Type of effect	Examples of pathologies/consequences
Metabolic effects	Type 2 diabetes mellitus (impaired glucose tolerance, insulin resistance)
	Cardiovascular disease, including contributory abnormalities: hypertension, dyslipidaemia, clotting defects
	Cancers (colon, breast, endometrium, kidney and oesophagus) – associated with upregulation of cell growth, or elevated hormone levels
	Hormonal dysfunction: menstrual abnormalities, pregnancy difficulties, anatomical changes
Mechanical effects	Musculoskeletal (including osteoarthritis in weight-bearing joints and back pain), resulting in disability
	Varicose veins, oedema
	Respiratory difficulties, including sleep apnoea and breathlessness
Surgical complications	Anaesthetic risk, poor wound healing, chest infections, thrombosis risk
Psychological/social effects	Tiredness, low self-esteem, depression, agoraphobia
	Family relationship problems, isolation
	Unemployment, discrimination

prevent cancer. There is, however, a lack of clear evidence to support mechanisms by which excess weight may cause cancer.

It is proposed that in obesity:

• Receptors for insulin-like growth factor (IGF) are upregulated, as a consequence of metabolic changes in response to insulin. Growth of cells, especially tumour cells, which utilise glucose, is promoted.

• Hormone-dependent cancers, such as those of the breast and prostate, are promoted due to the conversion of androgens to oestrogens in adipose tissue.

It is very difficult to separate the effects of obesity from those of dietary factors that may have contributed to the obesity, but at the same time also had a promoting effect on cancer development themselves. Nevertheless, weight loss and physical activity may be beneficial as preventive measures against cancer development in overweight subjects.

Other consequences of obesity

These are listed in Table 50.1, and relate to:

• the physical consequences of excessive weight on skeleton and joints;

• the consequences of increased effort by respiratory muscles required to overcome resistance in breathing;

• the consequences of higher body fat levels for anaesthesia, and ventilation during surgery;

• poor peripheral circulation, resulting in slower wound healing;

• social consequences of overweight and obesity in terms of societal perceptions, and effects on the formation and maintenance of personal relationships, if there is low self-esteem.

These have profound effects on the quality of life and the social experience of the affected individual, and may have serious implications for levels of morbidity.

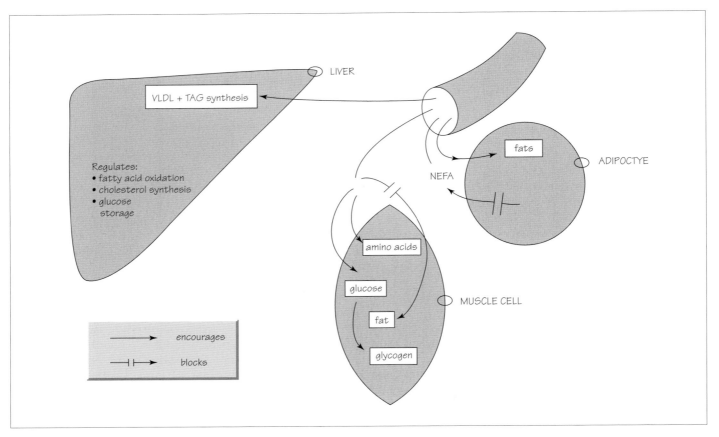

Fig. 51.1 Main actions of insulin under normal conditions.

Aims

(1) To consider insulin resistance as a major metabolic abnormality.
(2) To describe the metabolic syndrome and its diagnostic criteria.

Metabolic effects of obesity

Insulin resistance (and possibly glucose intolerance/type 2 diabetes), dyslipidaemia and hypertension are the major metabolic consequences of obesity. Their coexistence characterises the *metabolic*

Agreed criteria for diagnosis of metabolic syndrome

- Central obesity, with waist circumference above cut-off level for men (94 cm) and women (80 cm)) (European figures)

and **two** of the following:

- raised serum triglycerides (above 1.7 mmol/L);
- low HDL levels (below 1.03 or 1.29 mmol/L for men and women, respectively);
- systolic blood pressure above 130 mmHg, diastolic blood pressure above 85 mmHg, or treatment for hypertension;
- fasting plasma glucose above 5.6 mmol/L, or type 2 diabetes diagnosed.

Benefits of weight loss

It is estimated that a 10% weight loss can achieve:

Blood pressure: reduction by 10 mmHg.

Fasting blood glucose: reduction of up to 50% in newly diagnosed patients.

Insulin levels and sensitivity: 30% lower fasting insulin levels, 30% increase in sensitivity.

Progression to diabetes: 40–60% fewer developing diabetes.

Lipids: fall of 10% in total cholesterol, 15% in LDL cholesterol, 30% in TAGs, 8% increase in HDL cholesterol.

Mortality: 20% less from all causes, 30% less from diabetes-related disease.

syndrome (also known as insulin resistance syndrome or syndrome X). Generally the syndrome is prodromic for (i.e. leads on to) type 2 diabetes mellitus.

Insulin resistance

The normal function of insulin is to act overall as an anabolic hormone, by targeting a number of tissues, and either promoting storage of nutrients, or preventing their catabolism (Figure 51.1).

Features of insulin resistance

Mechanisms for insulin resistance have been studied extensively in animals, and findings include failure of second messenger signalling, presence of antagonists, a defect in a single cellular enzyme or cellular satiety due to overload with carbohydrate or fat.

However, in humans it appears that over 75% of insulin resistance is attributable to obesity and low physical fitness.

The key elements of the metabolic abnormality are shown in Figure 51.2, and can be summarised:

- Insulin resistance results in a *muted inhibition* of lipolysis of stored fat (**1**), with larger amounts of non-esterified fatty acids (NEFAs) released into the circulation. This is particularly detrimental in the visceral area, where the NEFAs arrive quickly in the liver via portal blood. It is for this reason that abdominal obesity is particularly involved.
- The NEFAs stimulate triacylglycerol (TAG) synthesis in the liver (**2**), and the *release of very low-density lipoproteins* (VLDLs) into the circulation.
- Elevated VLDLs exchange TAGs with high-density lipoproteins (HDLs) and low-density lipoproteins (LDLs), in exchange receiving cholesterol esters (**3**), producing small dense HDL (**4**).

- TAG-rich HDLs are broken down by hepatic lipase (**5**), resulting in a *reduction in levels of HDLs* in the circulation.
- TAG-rich LDLs also lose some of their TAGs in the liver by the action of hepatic lipase, becoming denser (**6**), due to a relative increase in the proportion of protein. These small dense LDLs are believed to be the most atherogenic lipoprotein particles, and thus contribute to increased CVD risk.
- Clearance of chylomicrons and VLDLs from the circulation is also reduced as activity of lipoprotein lipase (LPL) in adipose tissue is insulin dependent (**7**). Persistence of these lipoprotein fractions contributes to dyslipidaemia.
- The circulating fats are eventually deposited in tissues, resulting in pathological alterations. Deposits can occur in adipose tissue, in hepatocyctes and in skeletal muscle.

In addition to the above effects on fat metabolism, other consequences of insulin resistance include:

- High NEFA levels also inhibit glucose uptake and metabolism in tissues, resulting in *hyperglycaemia*. This in turn promotes increased insulin release, resulting in *hyperinsulinaemia*.
- Raised levels of insulin may independently activate sympathetic nervous system activity and the hypothalamic–pituitary axis, resulting in *hypertension*.

Insulin levels normally rise after meals as glucose concentrations rise, and are low in the postprandial state, when stored metabolites are used for energy.

When the response to insulin is muted, the condition is termed *insulin resistance*. In such subjects, a *higher plasma level of insulin is required* to achieve the same level of glycaemic control as in a normal subject.

Because insulin has a range of actions, resistance may affect all or only some of these, complicating the clinical picture.

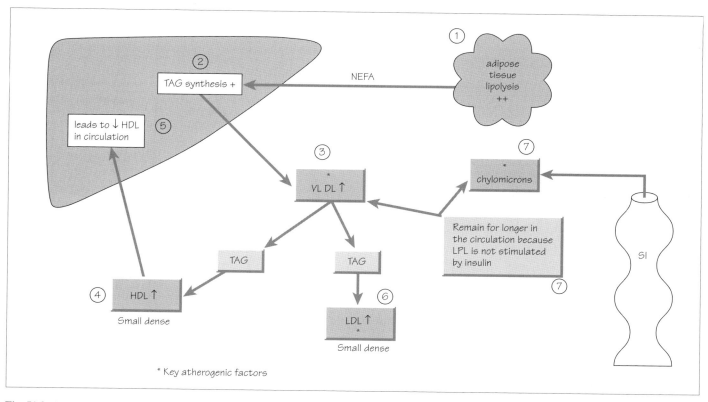

Fig. 51.2 Consequences of insulin resistance for fat metabolism.

52 Overweight and obesity: prevention and management

Aims

(1) To consider ways of preventing overweight and obesity.
(2) To describe options to achieve weight loss and its long-term management.

Prevention

Preventing an overweight individual from becoming obese should be easier, less expensive and more effective than tackling established obesity, where the magnitude of the weight loss required is greater. However, the impetus to tackle a weight problem may not be present at lower levels of overweight.

Obesity has a multifactorial aetiology (discussed in Chapter 49), which should be addressed at various levels (Table 52.1).

Despite a clear understanding of what needs to be done, these approaches have not achieved the expected success. Reasons might include:

- under-resourcing for individual action;
- inadequate monitoring of effectiveness;
- little surveillance to trigger early action on weight gain;
- insufficient coordination of initiatives.

Treatment

First-line treatment should be a *weight management programme,* whose goals are to:

- help overweight individuals lose weight;
- maintain this weight loss with appropriate changes to *lifestyle*

Behaviour change techniques

These include:

(1) Setting *realistic goals:* overambitious targets are likely to be demotivating. These may be weekly or monthly rates of loss, a percentage of current weight or simply stabilisation, with no further gain.

(2) *Support from family and friends:* may also occur by a group or programme leader and include support to overcome obstacles and setbacks.

(3) *Anticipating the barriers to progress:* may include keeping a diary to identify triggers to eating, coping with difficult situations and establishing self-belief for success.

and behaviour;

- achieve a reduction in risk factors.

These programmes may be offered in primary care, by local dietitians, commercial slimming groups and health clubs or freelance consultants offering 'lifestyle coaching'. There may be cost implications for clients, depending on the provider.

(For provision within the UK's National Health Service, referral may be prioritised on the basis of need, with those whose BMI is >30, or for a BMI below this level, with coexisting risk factors.)

A diet and lifestyle approach is used, combining:

- behaviour change;
- dietary measures;
- increased activity.

Drug treatment and surgery are only considered in more complex and severe cases (discussed below).

Dietary measures are based on healthy eating principles. These are discussed further in Chapter 53.

All dietary recommendations should be discussed with the individual and negotiated to take into account likes and dislikes, to maximise compliance. Additional help may include:

- shopping lists and menu plans;
- diet plans where counting calories for specific foods is the main focus;
- fat content may be counted or specific points allotted to foods.

These are all techniques that may help with compliance and will suit particular individuals, but not others.

There are also many other 'slimming diets' available for consumers, discussed in Chapter 53.

Activity provides an additional means of achieving a negative energy balance.

- In conjunction with dietary measures, activity contributes to weight loss, and protects the lean body mass. This helps to maintain the metabolic rate, which decreases when energy intake is reduced.
- Vigorous activity also results in a post-exercise elevation of metabolic rate, further enhancing energy utilisation.
- Activity can increase fat utilisation and sensitivity to insulin and improve blood lipid profiles.
- Activity induces a feeling of well-being, which can improve the mood and self-image of an individual on a weight loss programme.
- Increased mobility and lung function may be additional benefits.

Table 52.1 Approaches to prevention of overweight and obesity at the personal and societal levels.

Prevention at individual level	Prevention at community/policy level: action needed to facilitate individual change
Modify food choices to healthier balance	Policies on labelling/easy availability of healthier choices
Reduce total energy intake to match output: moderate portion sizes	Food industry action on smaller portions
Regulate snacking/choose healthier snacks/drinks	Limit advertising of less healthy snacks, especially to children
Engage in more physical activity, reduce sedentary activities	Encourage walking/cycling and sport by attention to the environment, transport policies, safety measures on roads and in urban spaces
Early awareness of a need for action on weight	Policy of monitoring weight in children; availability of health checks and accessible
Clear guidance on the health risks of excess weight and the need for change	evidence-based advice on weight management, with support
	Regulation of poor-quality/unsound advice

- Exercise on prescription, and referral to weight loss programmes and slimming groups, is becoming accepted within primary care.

Drug treatment

There are specific guidelines on the use of anti-obesity drugs. Three are currently available for use in the UK: orlistat, sibutramine and rimonabant (Table 52.2).

Individuals should also have appropriate advice on diet and physical activity with behavioural strategy support.

There are also a large number of over-the-counter formulations that claim to promote weight loss; none of these has been adequately evaluated for efficacy or safety.

Surgical treatment (bariatric surgery)

This is only used in cases of morbid obesity (BMI >40, or 35–40 where there are comorbidities). Two types of surgical intervention are used: malabsorptive and restrictive (Table 52.3).

The use of bariatric surgery in the UK is limited, but increasing. Appropriate follow-up arrangements must be available for patients to manage complications. Malabsorption conditions arising from bypass operations are associated with nutritional deficiencies and require supplementation.

Table 52.2 Overview of drugs currently licensed in the UK for weight loss.

	Orlistat	Sibutramine	Rimonabant
Mechanism of action	Inhibits fat digestion and absorption	Inhibits serotonin uptake in the brain; promotes satiety. May increase energy expenditure	Blocks cannabinoid receptors in the brain
Side effects	Fat appears in faeces, may cause faecal leakage	Adverse effects in hypertension	Mild and infrequent
Recommended for use	For people with BMI >30 (or >28 with diabetes, hypertension, raised cholesterol)	BMI >30, or >27 with comorbidities; not to be used for more than 12 months	Not currently used in depressed patients
Prior requirement	Should have managed some previous weight loss by diet/activity	Difficulty in achieving or maintaining weight loss	
Weight loss expected	5% at 3 months; 10% at 6 months	5% at 3 months	5–10% loss in 60–70% of patients
Long-term prospects	Maintenance of loss rarely achieved	Maintenance of loss rarely achieved	Maintained over 2 years; regained if drug stopped

Table 52.3 Overview of currently used surgical interventions for morbid obesity.

Name of treatment	Procedure	Comments
Malabsorptive surgery	Sections of GI tract bypassed to reduce surface area for absorption	Weight loss substantial and maintained. Metabolic complications include vomiting, stenosis, dumping syndrome. Patients need to be monitored
Jejuno-ileal	Bypasses a large area of small intestine (SI)	High risk of complications; rarely performed
Gastric bypass	Reduces stomach size and bypasses duodenum	Reduced capacity and digestion
Biliopancreatic diversion	As above, but jejunum also bypassed	More extensive effect on absorption
Restrictive surgery	Reduces the size of the stomach	Limits capacity for food, but not absorption
Gastroplasty	Stomach divided to make a smaller pouch (vertical division more successful)	Less weight loss than with gastric bypass
Gastric banding	Constricting band around stomach limits capacity, may be adjusted to vary extent of restriction	

53 Overweight and obesity: popular slimming diets

Aims

(1) To identify the criteria relating to a safe diet designed for weight loss.

(2) To consider the types of commercially available diets for weight loss.

The media promote 'diets', which are invariably focused on weight loss, such that the term 'diet' is synonymous in the public mind with eating less to achieve weight reduction. This is in contrast to the nutritionists' view, that 'diet' refers to an individual's food intake.

The slimming industry

For many people, a slow and steady weight loss seems unsatisfactory, and 'quick fix' regimes are sought. In addition, those who have regained weight may look for a new approach. As a result an ever-changing industry of slimming programmes has grown up to fill this need. A poorly balanced slimming regime may lead to nutritional deficiencies.

Principles of weight reduction

The scientific principle of weight reduction is apparently straightforward:

- energy intake must be less than energy output to create a negative energy balance, resulting in weight loss, as stored fat reserves are used for energy.
- energy deficits of 500–1000 kcal (2–4 MJ) per day may be recommended, depending on body size and gender.

Weight loss is generally slow, ~0.5 kg/week, unless the energy deficit is great, when there is also likely to be significant loss of lean tissue.

When weight has been lost, the further problem of *maintenance* creates a challenge to individuals, who may gradually regain weight, and so further 'dieting' is needed.

Criteria for a nutritionally sound and safe slimming regime

A slimming regime should fulfil a number of criteria (Table 53.1) in order to be considered sound.

Healthy eating guidelines can underpin dietary advice for weight loss in a number of ways. These are summarised in Table 53.2.

Types of slimming diets

Various approaches are used by the slimming industry, from ones that are safe and based on good principles, to others that can be viewed as potentially dangerous or at least misleading (Table 53.3).

1. Sensible healthy eating plans with reduced energy

A number of 'slimming' organisations have well-balanced diet plans, and use systems such as points or exchanges that allow the individual to adjust their intake in line with a target energy allowance. Some include an exercise regime and provide group support through regular meetings. Generally these are safe and meet essential criteria.

2. Diets that maintain satiety

The clear way to consume less energy is to eat less, but to ensure that this is acceptable, satiety needs to be maintained. This can be achieved by:

- Increasing intake of all plant foods. These can displace more energy-dense items, especially high-fat products, whilst providing bulk in the digestive tract, promoting satiety and avoiding hunger.

Table 53.1 Summary of criteria for a nutritionally sound and safe weight loss regime.

Criterion to be fulfilled	Explanation	Comment
Nutritionally balanced	No major food groups should be excluded or eaten to excess; principles that underpin healthy eating should be evident	Avoids risk of deficiency or need for supplements
Biologically plausible	Should not make claims that run against known biological facts	May be difficult for consumer to recognise
Safe	Must not recommend levels of intake that endanger health	Should carry advice to check with doctor
Realistic	Results promised should be realistic	Misleading claims will be demotivating
Flexible	Diet should allow some personal choices, to maintain motivation	Rigid eating regimes lead to abandonment
Sustainable	Diet should fit as much as possible into normal life; eating special and unusual foods may be a novelty, but does not fit easily into social existence	Special items increase costs and highlight 'dieting behaviour'
Physical activity	A sensible amount should be recommended to support dietary regime	Can improve self-image and help towards successful outcome

Table 53.2 Basic measures underpinning dietary advice for weight loss.

Dietary measure	Target change	Reasons for change/gain to be made
Reduction in total energy	2.4 MJ (600 kcal), or a 2–4-MJ (500–1000-kcal) deficit	To produce a negative energy balance
Lower total fat intake	To a moderate level	Monounsaturated fats should predominate
Starchy foods should be maintained	Include those with a lower glycaemic index	Maintain a steady blood glucose level, and avoid periodic hunger; a higher non-starch polysaccharide (NSP) intake will promote satiety
Fruit and vegetables	At least five a day	Provide micronutrients and low-energy, nutrient-dense intake. Useful snacks
Soft drinks	To be avoided	Provide energy and promote passive overconsumption

Table 53.3 Evaluating types of slimming diets against criteria.

Type of diet	Balanced	Plausible	Safe	Realistic	Flexible	Sustainable
Healthy eating plans	Yes	Yes	Yes	Yes	Yes	Yes
Increasing plant foods	Possible	Yes	Yes	Yes	Possible	Yes
Eating low-GI foods	Possible	Little evidence	Yes	Yes	Possible	Possible
Lower fat diets	Yes	Yes	Yes	Yes	Yes	If not too extreme
Low-CHO diets	No	No	No	No	No	No
Food combining	No	No	Possibly	Possibly	No	No
Eating at certain times	Possible	No	Possible	Possible	No	No
Preload before meals	Possible	No	No	No	No	No
Avoiding allergens	No	No	No	No	No	No
Supplement-requiring diets	No	No	No	No	No	No
Eating one food only	No	No	No	No	No	No
Fasting/meal skipping	No	No	No	No	No	No

This approach is used in many healthy diet plans, and provides a sound framework for weight loss.

• Eating foods with a lower glycaemic index (GI) in place of high-GI foods slows down the absorption of glucose and the release of insulin. It is suggested that the high levels of insulin promote fat storage, making high-GI foods more 'fattening'. At present there are insufficient data about the GI effect of mixed diets, as most studies have been done on single foods, so there is currently no evidence that this is a suitable diet to achieve weight loss.

3. Diets that adjust macronutrient content

Low-fat diets. Fat in the diet is more energy dense than other macronutrients, and is believed to be associated with 'passive overconsumption of energy', so reducing the intake of fat is a logical approach to follow. Many low-fat diets exist, where fat intake is 20–30% of total energy, with an increase in the content of complex carbohydrate.

This improves cardiovascular risk factors, and may protect from other chronic disease. Focusing on a reduction in fatty foods allows healthy eating to become established to help in longer term maintenance. Combining a reduction in the percentage of fat with an overall lowering of energy intake produces better weight loss than simply replacing fat with carbohydrate.

Low-carbohydrate diets. These have been promoted, with the energy being made up from protein and fat. The most famous of these is the 'Atkins diet'. There is initial rapid weight loss as glycogen reserves and the associated water are lost. The lack of carbohydrate for metabolism results in ketosis, which causes nausea, dehydration and bad breath. Constipation is likely because of the low fibre intake.

The high fat intake is contrary to all healthy eating principles. Weight loss does occur, but this is attributed to the anorectic effects of a high-protein diet, and the reduced overall energy intake. Low intakes of minerals and vitamins will, if not supplemented, result in deficiency.

4. Diets that prescribe meal composition or timing of meals

Food combining suggests that foods containing proteins should not be eaten with carbohydrate-containing foods, as they cannot be digested simultaneously. There is no scientific evidence for this. Weight may be lost because attention is being paid to what is eaten, and overall food intakes are likely to be reduced as a result.

Consuming foods only before a certain time in the day is proposed by another diet, to allow the body to complete digestion before night time. Again the main effect of this is to limit overall food intake.

5. Diets that 'preload' the digestive system before meals

Eating fruit before a meal to provide 'enzymes', or grapefruit to 'eliminate fat' are two suggested eating patterns, neither of which have any scientific base. In both cases, the preload is likely to reduce the food eaten at mealtimes.

Drinking water before meals to cause weight loss may promote a feeling of fullness at mealtimes and so reduce food intake. However, water is rapidly absorbed from the stomach, so would have a short-term effect.

6. Diets that avoid supposed 'allergic reactions'

These invoke claims that overweight is due to an allergic reaction by the body to food components that do not 'match', including eating different types of foods depending on blood group, or a mismatch of electric charges between the food and the individual. Both focus on elimination of entire food groups and are nutritionally dangerous without any scientific basis.

7. Diets that require supplements

A variety of these exist that are reported to boost energy, detoxify, improve cellular activity, etc. Unless there are clear medical reasons for poor digestion or absorption, these preparations will not help in weight loss.

8. Eating one food only

There are nutritionally balanced, single-item, very low energy diet products that can be used for short-term rapid weight loss. The popular diets that advise consuming a single product, such as cabbage soup, have no nutritional credibility, and are unsustainable.

Monotony and boredom restrict intake and the consumer learns nothing about a healthy balanced diet for future weight control. Serious risk of deficiency also exists.

9. Fasting/meal skipping

This may be seen as the easiest way of losing weight, but it is unsustainable, and likely to result in a very erratic food intake with the risk of nutritional deficiency. Risks of dehydration in the short term and eating disorders in the longer term are possible.

Weight loss needs to be addressed by a public health approach with a higher rate of success than at present; meanwhile vulnerable individuals will continue to be exposed to unsound and unsafe slimming regimes. It would be helpful if at least the awareness of what to look for in a weight reduction programme was more widely recognised.

Underweight and negative energy balance

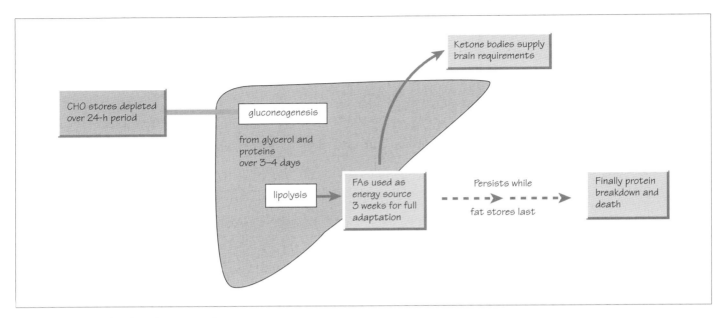

Fig. 54.1 Stages in the adaptation to starvation.

Aims

(1) To consider reasons for the development of underweight.

(2) To describe the body's response to a negative energy balance.

A deficit of energy intake, in naturally occurring situations (e.g. famine conditions), is generally accompanied by an inadequate intake of nutrients. There are a number of contributory factors, which may also determine the metabolic consequences and any treatment that is attempted.

The most obvious consequence of the energy deficit is *loss of weight*, attributable to an imbalance between energy intake (which is reduced) and energy expenditure (which may be increased, unchanged or even reduced from a previous level).

Causes of reduced energy intake

These might include:

- Poor food availability (this may be acute, as in a famine situation, or chronic, if food supplies are always poor, due to supply/crop production problems, or linked to a lack of assets).
- Inability to eat due to illness, or following injury or trauma.
- Intentional/deliberate restriction of food, either for a short term (e.g. to lose weight), or as a long-term behaviour (possibly associated with some form of eating disorder), or a political statement.

  Causes of increased energy expenditure might include:
- Heavy manual labour.
- Increased requirements for growth.
- Fever/infection/post-traumatic response.

In the majority of instances there is an *adaptive physiological response* to minimise energy expenditure when intake is reduced, and therefore facilitate survival. Adaptation may fail when there are other concurrent challenges to the body.

Starvation

This is the most challenging situation, as energy intake falls to zero.

When no food is eaten, the body must adapt to utilise stored energy reserves. The largest of these is body fat, stored in adipose tissue, which can supply fatty acids for energy provision. However, the brain and red blood cells require a supply of glucose to function, and metabolic adaptations must occur to preserve carbohydrate and use it efficiently.

Altogether, these adaptations allow savings to be made in energy output.

A number of neural and hormonal responses are involved; these include:

- reduced sympathetic nervous system activity;
- lower levels of active thyroid hormone (T_3);
- lower levels of insulin;
- leptin activity, which modulates the energy-sparing response.

Chronic energy deficits

For a large percentage of the population in the less developed countries, chronic energy deficiency is a permanent feature of their life. The adaptations that occur enable the body to survive, but often at a cost to long-term health (see Table 54.1).

Energy deficit compounded by disease or trauma

The concurrence of a metabolic response to disease or trauma with

Adaptation to starvation

This develops over a period of time, and involves changes to metabolism of substrates:

- Carbohydrate stores, as glycogen in liver and muscle, are limited, and may be completely exhausted within 24 hours.
- Hepatic gluconeogenesis can generate glucose *de novo*, from glycerol (from lipids) and carbon skeletons of amino acids. There is an initial phase, lasting 3–4 days, of protein breakdown from skeletal muscle for energy.
- A fall in circulating glucose and insulin levels stimulates lipolysis; tissues use more fatty acids for energy and glycerol is directed to gluconeogenesis. Ketone bodies are produced by the oxidation of fatty acids in the liver.
- The brain adapts to the use of ketone bodies for energy, meeting some two-thirds of its energy requirements in this way. Small amounts of glucose are produced by gluconeogenesis. This adapted steady state may take up to 3 weeks to establish, and can persist as long as fat reserves are available. This tends to be longer in women than in men, and depends on the previous level of nutrition. As women have more body fat, this extends the survival period.

- Once fat reserves are depleted, structural proteins are broken down, and there is a rapid deterioration leading to death. (See Figure 54.1 for a summary of this process.)

Adaptations of energy expenditure

These also occur, and therefore contribute to minimising the energy imbalance.

- Resting metabolism – there is an early phase of increased metabolic efficiency; later metabolism uses less energy as a result of a smaller mass of active tissue.
- Thermogenesis – where no food is consumed there will be no diet-induced thermic response; undernourished individuals have been shown to have a poorer thermogenic response on exposure to cold.
- Physical activity – observations of individuals who are starving, or in negative energy balance due to undernutrition, show that there is a reduced amount of physical activity undertaken. In addition there is a greater ergonomic efficiency in activity. The post-exercise elevation of heat output is also diminished in undernutrition.

Table 54.1 Adaptations to chronic energy deficits and their consequences.

Changes involving	Adaptation	Consequences for function/health
Body composition	Lower fat stores	Reduced resistance to cold
	Lower BMI; height and weight affected	Poorer growth and development
		Affects child-bearing capacity
		Poorly developed immune system and therefore resistance to infection
	Lower muscle mass, in relation to visceral development	Weaker respiratory muscles, tendency to chest infections
		Lower strength and work capacity, may perpetuate poverty
Energy expenditure	Less energy for work; more sedentary behaviour	Lower productivity/ability to engage in agricultural production
		Children engage less in play, affects social development
	Poorer response to injury	Longer time to recover from injury, poorer wound healing

energy deficit is likely to exacerbate the negative energy balance, for a number of reasons.

- Injury, infection and fever increase the metabolic rate, in proportion to the extent of the physiological stress.
- Protein is catabolised from muscle for the production of acute-phase proteins by the liver, and nitrogen losses increase.
- The major hormones of the stress response are cortisol and catecholamines, which stimulate glucose production and increase energy expenditure.

This metabolic response may result in a serious loss of weight in an undernourished patient which, together with tissue wasting and anorexia, results in cachexia, with a high risk of mortality. This can occur in some chronic illnesses. The need for nutritional support must be assessed and appropriate measures quickly introduced. This can be a major problem in hospital patients.

55 Nutrition and cancer I

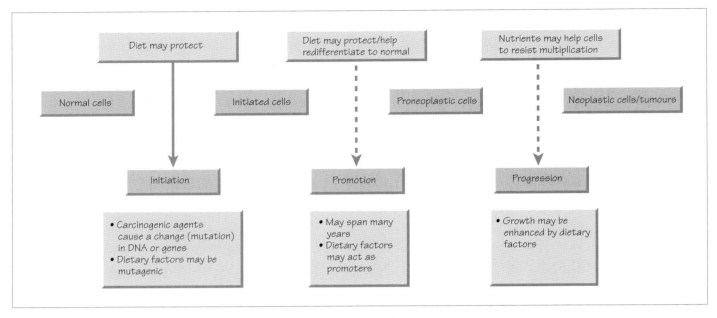

Fig. 55.1 Stages in the development of cancer and points at which diet may play a role.

Aims

(1) To consider the stages in the development of cancer where the diet may play a role.

(2) To describe the possible factors in the diet that may have a causative role in cancer.

Cancer is the cause of approximately one in four deaths in the UK and is a leading cause of mortality worldwide. Specific types of cancer vary in prevalence in different parts of the world (Table 55.1); this differential reflects the variety of environmental factors, including diet, that play a role in causation.

There is a growing burden of cancer deaths worldwide, associated with an ageing population. However, there are also differing trends in the rates of some cancers. For example, in the West lung cancer rates have been falling in men, but increasing in women, as smoking behaviours change. In Japan there has been a rapid increase in colorectal cancer rates during the last 30 years, as diets become more Westernised.

What is cancer?

Cancer is a disorder of somatic cells, in which changes to the genetic material cause a normal cell to behave abnormally in form or function. The change that occurs may be inherited, or occur sporadically. The result is that the cell fails to function as it should, in not responding to regulatory signals that control its life cycle. As a result it may divide inappropriately, or fail to die (apoptose) at the end of its life cycle, with the result that a cluster of cells is eventually produced, forming a tumour.

Stages in the development of cancer have been identified, and mechanisms within these are still being studied. However, it is clear that movement through the stages is not inevitable, and repairs can be made that stop or slow down the process.

It is within these 'accelerating' or 'braking' mechanisms that the environment and diet can play a role. These are summarised in Figure 55.1.

Evidence on causation of cancer

A number of environmental factors, including diet, have been associated with the aetiology of cancer. However, providing sound evidence is difficult.

• Much evidence is based on *epidemiological studies* of populations, allowing the calculation of the relative risk of the disease, based on levels of exposure to a causative factor. Epidemiology cannot provide proof of cause and effect, and associations may be confounded by other differences between populations. Studies of migrants who develop the rates of cancer typical of their host country within a generation, confirm the importance of environment.

• *Case-control studies* provide further information about exposure to causative factors, but the time course of cancer development can blur the relationship between exposure and diagnosis of cancer. Trials of interventions with putative preventive factors have been disappointing, and have failed to confirm the protective roles of

Table 55.1 Differences in prevalence of cancers in parts of the world.

Developed countries		Developing countries	
Men	*Women*	*Men*	*Women*
Lung	Breast	Lung	Breast
Prostate	Colorectum	Stomach	Cervix
Colorectum	Lung	Liver	Stomach
Stomach			

nutrients such as beta-carotene or vitamin E. Reasons for this may include the use of a single nutrient supplement rather than whole food sources, and timing of interventions.

• Very large-scale *prospective cohort studies* are now under way, such as the European Prospective Investigation of Cancer (EPIC), which has recruited over half a million participants who are being followed up, to identify cancer development and link this with earlier exposure to risk factors. Smaller cohort studies provide some evidence on diet and environmental associations, but with such homogeneous cohorts, there are limits to the general application of the results.

• Findings from population studies are gradually being tested in *experimental situations* to elucidate mechanisms. For example, an association between red meat intake and bowel cancer, observed by the EPIC study, has been tested experimentally. This has demonstrated that red meat consumption causes *N*-nitroso compound levels in faeces to increase, and that there is an increase in DNA mutations of colonic cells with higher levels of these compounds.

Diet as a factor in cancer

It is estimated that an average of 30% of cancer is diet related: this ranges from a low level for lung cancer, to 80% for colorectal cancer.

Difficulties in attributing causation to dietary factors occur because:

• diets are extremely complex, and particular nutrients can occur in many different foods;

• certain aspects of the diet co-vary in individuals, such that a high intake of one food, for example meat, may be associated with a low intake of fruit and vegetables;

• patterns of food intake obtained from food frequency questionnaires may not be sufficiently specific to demonstrate differences and relationships;

• dietary records may contain errors, but more robust techniques are being developed that cross-check dietary records with other markers.

Nevertheless, information about the roles of diet suggests that it can:

• be a source of preformed, or precursors of, carcinogens;

• contain nutrients that affect the formation, transport, deactivation or excretion of carcinogens;

• contain nutrients that can be protective, by promoting the body's resistance to carcinogens and the promotion of cancer.

Some evidence exists of a promoting effect of certain dietary factors in cancer (Table 55.2).

Avoidance of these foods or dietary components may help protect individuals against the development of cancer, and should feature in advice (see Chapter 56).

Table 55.2 Dietary factors that may have a role in promotion of cancer.

Food or nutrients	Possible role in cancer promotion
Total energy intake	High energy intakes promote rapid growth in children; this has been linked to a higher incidence of colorectal cancer later in life High energy intakes result in overweight and obesity, linked to greater incidence of hormone-related cancers: breast, endometrium and prostate. Also a positive association with cancers of: oesophagus, colorectum and kidney
Fat intakes	Difficult to separate from the evidence on overweight. High fat intakes (especially of saturated fat) have been associated with lung, colorectal, prostate and breast cancers There is little evidence of specific risk from monounsaturated or polyunsaturated fats. Conjugated linoleic acid (CLA), found in dairy fat, may have a protective role, but evidence is equivocal
Alcohol	May potentiate the role of other carcinogens, increasing uptake or susceptibility of cells Intakes linked with cancer of: aerodigestive tract and liver; also evidence of an association with breast cancer, possibly through an effect on oestrogen metabolism Some protection may be offered with adequate intake of folate
Salt	Linked with gastric cancer; high levels of salt reduce gastric acidity, which in turn promotes conversion of dietary nitrates to nitrites and nitrosamines, which are carcinogenic Better methods of preservation have reduced the use of salt for this purpose, and there has been a parallel reduction in gastric cancer
Meat	Metabolic products in the colon, arising from digestion of red meat are *N*-nitroso compounds, which have been found to cause DNA mutations. Thus there is a possible mechanism for development of colorectal cancer Processed meat and charred meat may also contribute by forming heterocyclic amines, which are broken down to carcinogenic products. Poultry and fish have not been associated with these changes

56 Nutrition and cancer II

Aims

(1) To describe possible factors in the diet that may have a protective role in cancer.
(2) To formulate dietary advice for prevention of cancer.

Protective effects against cancer can be obtained from foods and nutrients, which act to repair damage or prevent promotion and subsequent progression to tumour development (Table 56.1).

Summary of evidence on diet and cancer

Although conclusive evidence of cause and effect from dietary factors is largely lacking in the causation of cancer, there is a substantial body of evidence that points to relationships between dietary components and increased or reduced risk. It should also be recognised that maintenance of physical activity and not smoking are key lifestyle guidelines that should be adhered to. These are summarised in Table 56.2 for the commonest cancer sites.

There is evidence of a possible association for other sites and other dietary factors, but this at present is insufficient.

Advice on diet and lifestyle

The current evidence on cancer suggests that dietary change is important.

Following healthy eating guidelines, with particular attention to the following aspects, forms the cornerstone of dietary prevention of cancer:

- Maintenance of normal body weight.
- Physical activity according to guidelines (at least 30 minutes on five days per week).
- At least 400 g/day of fruit and vegetables, including a variety of

Table 56.1 Dietary factors with a possible protective role in cancer.

Food or nutrients	Possible role in protection against cancer
Non-starch polysaccharides (dietary fibre)	Diets high in fibre confer some protection against colorectal cancer This may be effected in a number of ways: –more rapid removal of potential carcinogens by faster transit through the bowel –more beneficial nutrients available for the colonocytes –healthier bacterial flora in a more acidic environment However, fibre intakes show high covariance with other beneficial foods, such as cereals, grains, fruit and vegetables, which may also have beneficial effects in other ways
Fruit and vegetables	There is consistent evidence that diets high in fruit and vegetables are associated with lower cancer rates, and no evidence to the contrary It is believed that the antioxidants supplied by these foods play a protective role against damage to DNA and other molecules. Firm evidence of this is lacking, however Other substances contained in fruit and vegetables may be important: these include various phytochemicals such as flavonoids, phytosterols, isothiocyanates, sulphur-containing compounds and phyto-oestrogens. A wide range of fruit and vegetables must be eaten to incorporate all of these
Folic acid	Some evidence suggests that higher intakes of folate are associated with lower risk of cancer, particularly of the colon, cervix, lung, breast and prostate; the mechanism appears to be a protection against mutations of DNA
Calcium and vitamin D	An inverse relationship between calcium intake (as dairy products) and colon cancer has been reported This may be due to binding in the gut of fats by calcium, thus reducing potential harm from fats and bile acids Vitamin D may have an anti-cancer action in its own right, and has been proposed to reduce risk of prostate, colon and breast cancer

Table 56.2 Summary of dietary factors for which there is strong or convincing evidence of a role in causation or protection against cancer.

Cancer site	Convincing/probable evidence of protection	Convincing/probable evidence of causation
Aerodigestive system	Fruit and vegetables	Alcohol, smoking, tobacco
Stomach	Fruit, vegetables, vitamin C sources, refrigeration	Salting of food for preservation
Colorectum	Vegetables, folate, fibre, calcium and vitamin D; physical activity	Overweight/obesity, red and processed meat, total fat
Liver		Alcohol, aflatoxins
Lung	Fruit, vegetables	Smoking
Breast	Fruit, vegetables	Alcohol, obesity, fat intakes

types.
• Increased intake of plant foods rich in complex carbohydrates, e.g. grains, cereals and pulses, to provide main source of energy.
• Minimal alcohol consumption.

• Reduced intakes of red meat, fat and salt.
• Avoidance of salt-preserved and processed foods.
• Safe food preparation: avoidance of foods that are spoilt or potentially contaminated with moulds, etc.

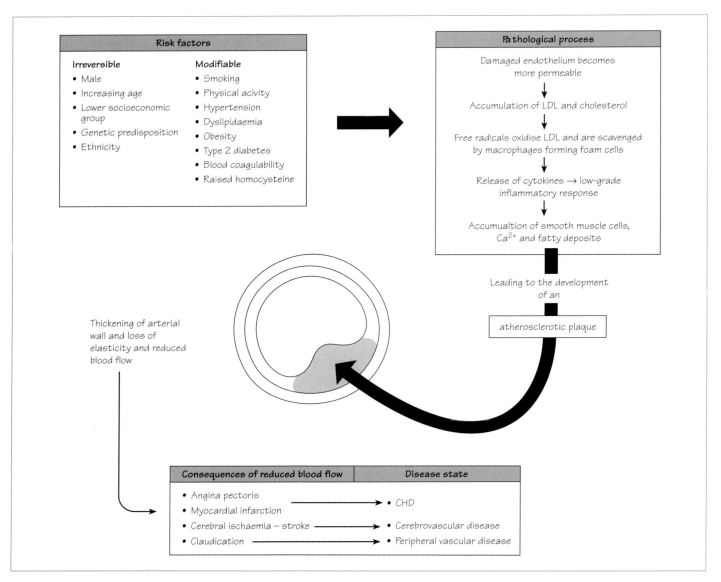

Fig. 57.1 Summary of the risk factors, pathological process and consequences of the atherogenic process.

Aims

(1) To describe the development of cardiovascular disease.
(2) To identify the major risk factors involved in the aetiology of the disease.

Mortality rates

Cardiovascular disease is the leading cause of death in the UK and accounts for approximately one-third of all deaths worldwide (almost 20 million annually). CHD deaths comprise about half of the total and stroke deaths a further quarter.

• Death rates due to CVD vary worldwide; in general rates are higher in industrialised countries, but with substantial variation.

Definitions

Cardiovascular disease (CVD) includes coronary heart disease (CHD), cerebrovascular disease and peripheral vascular disease (PVD). All share the common features of thickening and hardening of the arterial walls resulting in a compromised blood flow.

• Highest rates are currently in Eastern Europe and lower in Japan and Mediterranean countries.
• Developing countries are experiencing rapid increases in these diseases as they undergo economic and nutritional transition; rates have been falling in many Westernised countries.

Pathology

The fundamental lesion is the atherosclerotic plaque that develops within the arterial wall and its eventual rupture. These processes occur slowly and over a prolonged period.

Three main stages can be described, summarised in Figure 57.1.

(1) The *vascular endothelium* is the key surface at which several contributory factors interact. The endothelium has many self-regulating properties, achieved through the production of nitric oxide, prostacyclin and other bioactive substances. Many of the risk factors cause dysfunction here. As a consequence, the endothelium becomes more permeable to lipids and proteins.

(2) *Low-density lipoproteins* (LDL) in the blood readily pass into the arterial wall to deliver cholesterol to the tissues. If they become oxidised, the cascade of events results in the formation of atherosclerotic plaque.

(3) If the *plaque becomes unstable and ruptures*, activation of platelets and the coagulation cascade can result in *thrombosis* and a myocardial infarction (or ischaemic stroke in the case of its occurrence in the brain).

Risk factors for CVD

The pathological process comprises many elements, which may be exacerbated or ameliorated by 'risk factors'.

Two categories are identified: *irreversible* and *potentially modifiable* (behavioural) (see Figure 57.2).

Irreversible risk factors

- Genetic traits – include disorders of lipid metabolism.
- Male gender – higher risk than in premenopausal women; risk equalises later in life.
- Increasing age – progressive increase of risk.
- Lower socioeconomic status – associated with higher risk.
- Ethnicity – higher risk in some ethnic groups (e.g. from Indian subcontinent).
- Small for gestational age at birth – greater risk in later life.

Modifiable (behavioural) risk factors

These are related to diet and lifestyle factors, and have been the focus of health education initiatives for many years. Many of the above risk factors overlap, either in their consequences, or in the causative factors (Figure 57.2).

Many of the risk factors have dietary components which contribute to or minimise the diesease process. These are discussed further in Chapter 58.

- *Smoking* – contributes to endothelial dysfunction and increases oxidative stress, promoting oxidation of LDLs.
- *Physical activity* – an increased level of activity reduces the impact of many other risk factors: physical activity reduces obesity, which is associated with insulin resistance, hypertension and abnormal blood lipids; lipid profiles are normalised, including an increase in HDL levels; endothelial function and clotting-related factors are improved; markers of inflammation decrease.

The modifiable risk factors offer an opportunity for intervention by health professionals, both as general health education or as targeted individual advice, to reduce the eventual risk of developing CVD. If CVD is already present, then more intensive advice or secondary prevention may be necessary.

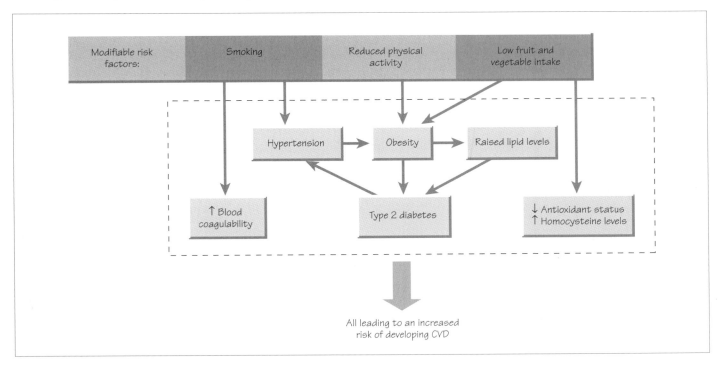

Fig. 57.2 Interactions between the major modifiable risk factors for CVD.

Aims

(1) To describe the evidence for the dietary factors involved in each stage of the development of cardiovascular disease.
(2) To use this evidence to formulate practical dietary advice.

The aetiology of cardiovascular disease (CVD) is multifactorial, with a number of risk factors influencing the development and progression of the disease.

From an understanding of the pathology of CVD (see Chapter 57), it is possible to identify dietary components that either contribute to or help to prevent the disease process. Although incomplete, current knowledge is used to advise on diets that reduce CVD risk.

Endothelial dysfunction

There is no 'gold standard' measurement for endothelial function, but vasodilatory capacity and assay of endothelium-derived products in plasma and urine are used as proxy indicators of function.

Many of the factors that affect the endothelium (see Table 58.1) also influence other stages of the pathological process.

Blood lipids

The *quantity* and *composition of dietary fats* are recognised as key determinants of the plasma lipid profile.
- Persistently elevated triglyceride levels alter the normal exchange of constituents between lipoprotein fractions (see Chapter 16) resulting in the formation of small dense LDLs and HDLs, which promote atherogenesis.
- Modifications to the proportions of consumed fats have been at the core of advice regarding dietary prevention of CHD since the 1970s.

The goals are to achieve *reductions in total cholesterol*, particularly that in the LDL fraction, and an *increase in HDL levels*. This advice reflects developments in knowledge, and is summarised in Table 58.2.

Oxidative stress

The *oxidation of LDL particles* is a key stage in the pathology of cardiovascular disease. LDL particles contain large amounts of polyunsaturated fats, which are vulnerable to oxidation. Markers of oxidative stress are increased in cardiovascular disease.

Other dietary factors impacting lipids

Other foods and nutrients that have been associated with effects on blood lipids, include:
- *Soya*: Isoflavones are able to reduce plasma cholesterol. A reduction of 0.23 mmol/L with an intake of 25 g soya protein/day has been reported.
- *Dietary fibre*: Soluble fibre has been reported to reduce total cholesterol by 0.045 mmol/L for each gram of fibre. Population studies suggest that lower rates of CHD are associated with larger intakes of dietary fibre.
- *Alcohol*: Moderate intakes of alcohol (1–2 units per day) have been shown to reduce CHD in men (above 40 years) and post-menopausal women. Levels of HDLs are increased, but greater consumption increases TAGs and CHD risk.
- *Plant stanols and sterols*: These reduce the absorption of dietary cholesterol and may also increase the activity of the LDL receptor; have a clear effect on reducing plasma cholesterol levels, especially in the LDL fraction.

Antioxidants are also present within the LDLs, and can provide some protection against free radicals. The diet is an important source of exogenous antioxidants.
- *Fruit and vegetables* are the main dietary sources of antioxidants, and populations in which there is a high level of consumption of these foods have a reduced risk of cardiovascular disease. An inverse association has been shown between plasma levels of antioxidants, including ascorbate and vitamin E, and cardiovascular disease risk.
- Intervention trials, using individual *antioxidant vitamins* alone or in combination, have failed to show evidence of benefit, and in some cases produced negative outcomes.
- Plant foods contain other compounds with antioxidant activity such as the *flavonoids*, and some of these may be the more active antioxidants when the whole foods are eaten. Current advice is to increase consumption of fruit and vegetables to at least five portions (or 400 g) per day, thereby providing a range of antioxidants.

Table 58.1 Factors involved in endothelial function.

Factor	Suggested mechanism	Strength of the evidence
Dietary fat intake	Elevated levels of TAG-rich lipoproteins, after meals have a pro-oxidant effect on the endothelium, may impair vasodilation	Consistent for harmful effect of atherogenic lipaemia
Fish oils	Especially docosahexaenoic acid (DHA), incorporated into membrane phospholipids, attenuates proinflammatory and prothrombotic activity	Evidence is consistent for reduction in fatal CHD
Antioxidant nutrients	Protect against free-radical damage, e.g. resulting from hypertension, smoking and pro-oxidant products	Consistent evidence from laboratory and *in vivo* studies; benefits not shown in intervention trials
B vitamins and folate	Reduction of homocysteine (HCys) levels in circulation. HCys is believed toxic to endothelium, possibly through reduced response to acetylcholine	Reduction in vascular events in treatment groups and improved ECG; large trials of supplementation awaited
Alcohol	Increases HDL levels, which act as antioxidants. May also have anti-inflammatory effect	Moderate intakes lower CHD

Table 58.2 Practical advice on dietary fats to modify plasma lipids and the origins of such advice.

Dietary lipid	Effect on plasma lipids	Practical application
Total fat	High-fat diets generally associated with high CHD rates. Low-fat diets are shown to reduce LDL levels. However, replacement of fat with CHO may increase TAG levels; the effect can be counteracted with physical activity	Fat reduction to 30–35% of total energy is widely recommended. More substantial reduction may limit compliance, and may result in high CHO intakes, which increase VLDL levels
SFAs	SFAs with 14 and 16 carbons are particularly strongly related to raised LDL levels. Reduction in SFA intake reduces total cholesterol, LDL and HDL (less than LDL); effects on CHD well supported with evidence	Reductions in dietary sources of SFA generally agreed; target intakes normally 10% of total energy
Cholesterol	Increases levels of plasma cholesterol to varying extent in individuals. Absorption from diet is limited	Closely associated with SFA in the diet, and emphasis on reducing SFA also limits intake of cholesterol. Eggs are cholesterol rich and intake may need to be controlled in susceptible individuals
n-6 PUFAs	Replacement of SFAs with n-6 PUFAs reduces LDL levels, with little change to HDL levels, resulting in improved lipid profile. May also help clearance of VLDLs in postprandial state	Substitution of SFAs with n-6 PUFAs recommended. Intakes above 10% of energy not recommended due to risk of peroxidation of double bonds
MUFAs	Replacement of SFAs with MUFAs reduces LDL levels, but not HDLs. Habituation to higher MUFA intake is associated with larger chylomicrons, and attenuated factor VII activation (i.e. lower blood clotting tendency)	Substitution of SFAs with MUFAs is a beneficial dietary modification, especially in subjects with normal body weight where total fat reduction is unnecessary
Trans fatty acids	Cause an increase in LDLs and reduce HDL levels, potential to contribute to CHD	Levels should be kept low; <2% of energy intake is recommended
n-3 PUFAs	Reported to improve the clearance of VLDLs from circulation and lower concentrations of small, dense LDLs	Effects on lipid clearance seen at high doses only, greater than can be achieved with acceptable intakes from oily fish

Inflammation

An inflammatory state appears to exist in cardiovascular disease, probably resulting from a generalised response to local factors associated with the atherosclerotic plaque.

Key indicators of this response are raised levels of C-reactive protein (CRP) and fibrinogen.

• *Obesity* is associated with raised levels of CRP, and levels fall on weight loss. However, it is unclear how and to what extent these findings are related to the inflammatory response.

• *Eicosanoids* derived from PUFAs play a part in inflammation, and those from the *n-6 PUFAs are pro-inflammatory*. Their synthesis is competitively inhibited by EPA and DHA present in oily fish, and the eicosanoids produced by the *n-3 PUFAs may be anti-inflammatory*.

• Additional effects of n-3 PUFAs may include increased plaque stability and altered cytokine production. However, at present it remains unclear how the n-3 PUFAs exert the documented protective effect in cardiovascular disease.

Haemostatic factors

The balance between *clotting tendency* and *fibrinolysis* determines the risk of thrombus formation. A large number of physiological factors have a role in these processes.

• *Obesity* has been associated with a raised concentration of fibrinogen and other markers of prothrombotic tendency. Weight loss and physical activity have a positive effect on these markers. Some of the contributors to a high energy intake may also affect thrombotic state; e.g. heavy alcohol consumption and a high-fat diet both reduce fibrinolytic activity. However, moderate alcohol intakes may reduce fibrinogen concentration.

• Fibrinolytic activity is also improved by diets that promote weight loss, such as low-fat and high-fibre diets.

• *Fish oils, providing n-3 PUFAs,* attenuate the production of thomboxane A_2 and so suppress activation of platelets.

Conclusions

Taking all the stages of the pathological process individually enables a detailed breakdown of the associated dietary factors to be considered. However, many factors have effects across several components of the process, and these form the basis of dietary advice for prevention of cardiovascular disease.

Key dietary aspects

• Moderate total fat intake.
• Replace the saturated fats with polyunsaturated fats or preferably monounsaturated fats.
• Increase intake of n-3 polyunsaturated fats, preferably from oily fish.
• Consume at least five portions of fruit and vegetables per day.
• Eat whole-grain products to increase dietary fibre intake and provide additional micronutrients.
• If alcohol is included, consume in moderate amount only.
• Maintain healthy body weight and remain physically active.

Aims

(1) To consider the concept of optimal nutrition.
(2) To consider different ways in which optimal nutrition might be achieved.

Advances in nutritional knowledge have led to an awareness that:
- there is *a minimal* quantity of a nutrient required to fulfil its physiological role;
- *amounts greater than this* can maintain normal function in health and provide a reserve against inadequate intakes or greater needs;
- *intakes above these levels* may operate in non-nutritional, or protective ways;
- *other factors* in foods, which do not have a clear nutritional role, may be *beneficial to health*.

Thus the concept of nutritional adequacy can cover a spectrum from 'preventing deficiency' to 'optimal nutrition'.

Some populations in the world have inadequate access to food for reasons such as low income or poor availability, and may not reach nutritional adequacy.

At the other end of the spectrum, in the richer countries, food industries provide a constantly expanding range of special products that aim to optimise health through nutrition.

Balanced diet

The concept of a balanced diet was discussed in Chapter 8.

In essence, the balanced diet is constructed using *major food groups*, and the main nutrients that they supply. These are quantified into numbers of servings so that the individual consumes a mixture of foods, and therefore nutrients, that meet dietary goals.

Optimal nutrition

The recognition that there are dietary links in the aetiology of many diseases has led to the concept of optimal nutritional status.

For a dietary constituent this is the level of intake required for:
- the maintenance of good health;
- reduction of chronic disease risk;
- prevention of overt nutritional deficiency and associated health risk.

Many foods are promoted as being beneficial for health, and this can lead to confusion for consumers who want clear advice about their health benefits.

Achieving optimal nutrition

Approaches that could result in improvements to nutritional status include:

Preventing deficiency

The concepts of Requirements and Dietary Reference Values are discussed in Chapter 7. Figures published in Recommended Intake tables provide the scientific basis on which nutrient-based guidelines and dietary goals are formulated.

In *practical terms*, it is easier for consumers to relate to *food-based guidelines*, which therefore form the basis of advice about balanced diets.

- supplementary feeding;
- fortification of specific food commodities;
- introduction of 'functional foods' into the diet.

It should also be noted that changes in nutritional behaviour can be brought about through approaches that change knowledge, skills and attitudes.

Supplementary feeding

Vulnerable groups in the population may be targeted with a specific supplementary feeding programme, on the basis of an assessed need.

This may be achieved through:
- a *balanced* supplement containing macro- and micronutrients; or
- one containing a particular micronutrient that had been found to be lacking (most frequently iron).

Most commonly used with vulnerable groups (such as pregnant women, children) in situations of undernutrition or disrupted food supplies, the *effectiveness* of this type of programme is *difficult to evaluate*.

Fortification of foods

The addition of a nutrient or nutrients to a widely consumed food can target a whole population group. Issues to consider include the choice of nutrient, the vehicle used for fortification, its acceptability and costs.

Many food products are fortified, either by law or by choice of the manufacturer. Examples include:
- White flour, bread and margarine are fortified by law in the UK.
- Other products that may be fortified in other countries include salt (with iodine), milk (with vitamin D) and flour (with folate).
- In the UK there is *voluntary fortification* of breakfast cereals, some dairy products (including yogurts and milk), infant foods, bedtime drinks and fruit juices.

There is a growing trend towards the production of fortified foods that promise the consumer protection against disease, such as osteo-

Quantifying optimal nutrition

At present, information about optimal levels of nutrients is incomplete, with more research needed about both individual influences and nutrient functions, including:
- what is the functional bioavailability of a nutrient?
- what is the key marker of nutrient *status*, sensitive to changes in intake?
- what is the key marker of nutrient *function,* sensitive to changes in status?

There are many factors that may influence the above, related to:
- *individual variability* (genetic, ethnicity, environment, social factors, age);
- different *responses at certain life stages* and how these can lead to disease;
- *interaction* between dietary constituents, affecting their bioavailability (including nutritional and non-nutritional components).

Reduced-nutrient foods

Some foods may have a reduced content of a nutrient.
- Lower fat or lower sugar products to achieve a 'low calorie' content, although the overall reduction in energy may not be very great.
- Low-salt foods may be formulated to reduce the content of sodium.
- There are also special products that cater for consumers requiring products low in lactose, milk-free, gluten-free, etc.

porosis, heart disease and cancer, and containing a range of minerals or vitamins.

The *impact of fortification* on nutritional status depends on the degree of 'saturation' with the fortified product. If alternatives are available, then the effectiveness will be reduced.

Points to consider include:
- The addition of folate to flour has in the USA resulted in a measurable reduction in the incidence of neural tube defects in fetuses.
- Iodisation of salt is an important public health measure that succeeds in reducing the incidence of goitre and cretinism.
- Even with a choice of products available, fortification of a relatively common product, such as breakfast cereal, can raise the nutritional status across a range of nutrients, of vulnerable groups, such as older adults.

Functional foods

This term covers a wide range of products that carry the common claim of possessing some health-promoting properties. This could be applied to many normal foods, but is more specifically used to describe foods that are rich in non-nutritional factors that are either naturally present, or have been added to achieve a possible health benefit (Table 59.1).

Organic foods

Consumers generally believe that foods produced organically, often by more traditional agricultural methods, have superior nutritional quality. This is not currently supported by the scientific literature, in which studies find no difference in nutrient content between organic and non-organic produce; there is also no information about impact on human health. It is, however, probable that organic foods contain little or no residual levels of pesticides and herbicides.

At the present time, organic food is more expensive and this may mitigate against consumption of an adequate diverse diet. It is preferable therefore to ensure adequate intake of a balanced diet, even if this is not organically produced. There is more evidence supporting the need for a good healthful range of foods than for the benefits of organic food.

Other dietary supplements

There is a wide diversity of supplements on the market, some derived from common foods, others from plants that are not normally consumed as part of the diet. Although they may be perceived by consumers as enhancing nutritional status, this can only be the case when the supplement taken is a nutrient. In all other cases, the effect is non-nutritional.

These non-nutritional supplements may be taken to:
- prevent or treat diseases that are not the result of deficiency (e.g. menstrual symptoms, prevention of a cold, stimulate the immune system, protect the liver, increase mental alertness, relieve arthritic pain);
- enhance sporting performance (e.g. ergogenic aids, muscle-building products, body shaping products).

In both cases, the evidence is generally weak and not supported by clinical trials.

Table 59.1 Examples of functional foods.

Product grouping	Examples	Sources	Possible function
Non-nutritional factors naturally present in foods			
Terpenoids	Carotenoids, including β-carotene, lutein, lycopene	Carrots, green leafy vegetables, orange- and red-coloured fruits and vegetables	Antioxidant role
Phenolic compounds, especially flavonoids and isoflavones	*Flavonoids:* Quercetin Catechins Anthocyanins	Apples and onions Tea and red wine Red/purple fruits and berries	Antioxidant role
	Isoflavones: Genistein Daidzein (termed phyto-oestrogens)	Soya and its products	Hormonal effects (probable oestrogenic/antioestrogenic effect), cholesterol-lowering effect
Glucosinolates	Isothiocyanates	Brassica family of vegetables	Possible anticancer role
Non-nutritional factors added to foods			
Phytosterols and stanols	β-Sitosterol, campesterol	Plant foods; derived from wood pulp and paper industry byproducts Added to margarines and some dairy foods	Cholesterol-lowering effect
Prebiotics and probiotics			
Beneficial bacteria and food sources for them	Lactobacilli, bifidobacteria; prebiotics may contain oligosaccharides	Dairy products, including yogurts, supply *probiotics. Prebiotics* may be included in infant formula, bakery products	Normalise gut bacteria; reduce growth of pathogenic organisms. Regulate bowel function; modify allergic responses, increase immunity

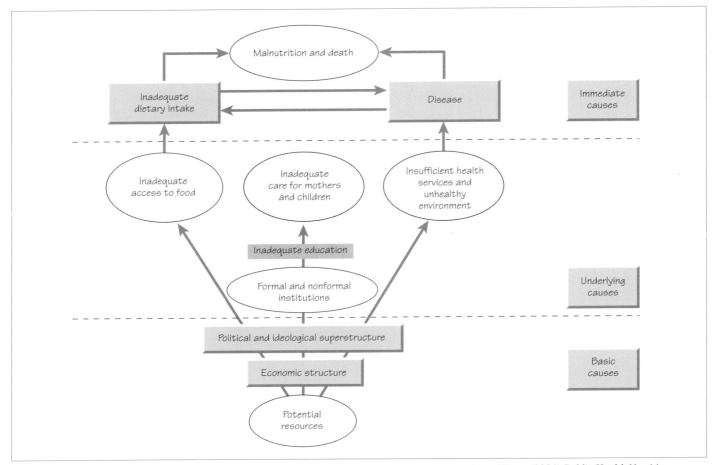

Fig. 60.1 United Nations Children's Fund (UNICEF) conceptual model (reproduced with permission from Gibney (2004) *Public Health Nutrition*, Blackwell Publishing).

Aims

(1) To recognise the multiple causes of poor nutrition.

(2) To describe the stages involved in developing a public health programme.

In order that people maximise their achievement of nutritional health, and so prevent disease and prolong life, scientific knowledge about nutrition should permeate all levels of a society.

This can be seen as the *public health nutrition approach,* which focuses on the promotion of good health throughout the population. In doing this, it uses a *biological and social science base*, together with a foundation of *epidemiology* and a *health promotion* approach.

In this way public health nutrition aims to engage all levels of society in promoting health and prolonging life.

UNICEF model of causation of malnutrition (Figure 60.1)

It is essential to recognise that health is more than the absence of disease, but rather encompasses:

- both physical and mental health; and
- the ability of people to make choices to enable these to occur.

Therefore the societal framework is important, together with the policies that exist to shape it.

UNICEF has developed a model that is widely used, and demonstrates how disease and poor nutrition are the result not simply of the immediate food supply, but reflect a number of *underlying causes* related to access to food, education and health care, in addition to more *basic structural causes* in a society, which include economic and political structures. Therefore making changes to the food intake necessitates *engagement at all of these levels in society* if the solutions are to be long lasting.

Aim of public health nutrition

Public health nutrition aims to find solutions to problems, whereby health will be improved. In order to reach this outcome, several logical stages must be completed.

1. Identify the problems

At the outset, it is necessary to identify the problems, and their links with nutrition. This requires:

• *Data on the prevalence and incidence of disease*, patterns of morbidity and mortality and profiles of groups affected. This information may be collected routinely by health surveillance, but its accuracy and penetration may vary. An independent nutritional assessment may be needed to establish this baseline information.

• *Scientific evidence*, based on a critical appraisal of the literature that the problems identified have a plausible nutritional link. This may be based on previous epidemiological studies.

• *Food intake patterns* from the population need to be identified as supporting the role of particular aspects of the intake in the nutritional problem. There should be a realistic assessment of the feasibility of altering these intakes to a more desirable level.

• *The constraints* that operate within the population should be identified, so that any goals and targets take these into account.

2. Broad aims and goals

For any public health intervention it is essential to set broad aims and goals, in order that a specific improvement can be assessed against the baseline, to evaluate the effectiveness of the intervention.

The broad aims may be part of a general policy, for example to reduce the incidence of coronary heart disease over a period of time.

3. Clear objectives

Clear objectives must be established. There may be nutritional as well as other objectives, for example relating to physical activity or food provision. Nutritional objectives may relate, for example, to the consumption of fruit and vegetables in the population.

4. Quantifiable targets

From the objectives, quantifiable targets should be set: for example, this might include a change in the sales of fruit and vegetables by supermarkets.

Any change must be measured against the baseline level, so tools to do this have to be available from the outset. The targets set should be *specific, measurable, realistic* and *achievable*, as well as *worthwhile* for the overall aim. The time frame in which they are to be achieved must be clear.

5. Planning the programme

Once the aims have been refined into measurable targets, the programme can be planned in such a way that the targets can be achieved.

In aiming to alter the intake of specific food(s), the planning needs to consider all of the factors that apply to the current level of intake, and whether there is potential to change these. Consideration may need to be given here to:

• the basic *factors affecting food intake*, such as the economic situation, or the political support for increasing the intake;

• underlying factors such as the *level of education* of the main food purchasers, and the potential to promote an increase through education;

• an *awareness* or a *desire for change*;

• other forces, such as advertising, or other *sectors with different interests*, e.g. commercial pressures from within the food industry, may be opposing factors.

Programmes may be *aimed at different levels*, or a combination of levels. They may target:

• basic factors, e.g. through government policy, e.g. on standards for school meals;

• underlying factors, e.g. by providing information on food labels to inform about the 'healthiness' of foods, or running cooking skills classes to enable people to take more control of their food intake options;

• promotion of specific foods, such as fruit and vegetables with targeted supermarket campaigns, school fruit schemes.

These approaches may be *combined* in an attempt, for example, to increase fruit and vegetable intake:

• school meals standards include a requirement to serve fruit and vegetables at each meal;

• cooking skills for preparation of vegetables and fruit;

• the introduction of children to fruit in school.

6. Implementing the programme

The final decision on implementing the programme may need to be pragmatic, in terms of:

• anticipated effectiveness (based on previous knowledge);

• feasibility;

• acceptability to the target population (or individuals);

• cost.

Costs of all the stages of the project must be mapped.

Timescales for achievement of intermediate stages in the project help to ensure the work remains on track, and to allow achievement of targets and evaluation of the activity by the end date.

7. Evaluation

This assesses both the process (i.e. the delivery of the programme) and the impact (i.e. to what extent did it achieve its goals).

The whole process of public health nutrition intervention tends to be *cyclical*, so that the evaluation of one programme generally leads to identification of further problems that can be addressed by a subsequent programme.

Programmes may be affected by external factors, outside their control, which may have positive or negative influences on outcomes. These need to be taken into account in any evaluation (see Chapter 61).

61 Promoting nutritional health: a public health perspective II

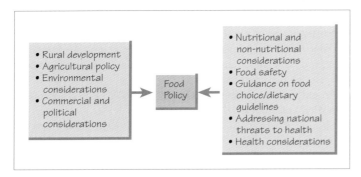

Fig. 61.1 Factors determining food policy.

Aims

(1) To identify the barriers to implementing successful dietary change.

(2) To describe the relationship between food and nutrition policy and public health nutrition.

Barriers to successful dietary change

In implementing public health nutrition programmes, outcomes may be poorer than expected. This may be attributed to a number of possible barriers.

Even with the best planned public health nutrition programmes, health intervention may fail to make an impact on diet and produce no measurable change in dietary habits. This can occur at any of the stages of the process:

(1) The intended subject **does not receive the message**: this may be because the medium for transmitting the message was inappropriate for the particular subject group. Identifying the most suitable channels of communication is an essential part of the planning process.

(2) The message **did not attract the attention** of the target subject group: this may be because it was not articulated in the most appropriate way to catch attention or to maintain interest throughout the delivery (either written, audio or oral).

(3) The message was **not correctly understood** – either misinterpreted and incorrectly followed, or simply pitched at a level inappropriate for the capabilities of the subjects. Appropriate piloting of the messages should ensure that these are understood.

(4) The subject finds the **message too complicated**, forgets the information or does not believe the information, if perhaps it contradicts commonly held beliefs in their culture, or is not delivered in a way that inspires belief.

(5) The message is received and understood, but does not result in behaviour change because of **other constraints**, for example income, or availability or attractiveness of the food changes to be made.

(6) Although the information received is acted on, it **does not bring about the expected changes in health**.

Unsuccessful health promotion activities may in themselves produce a negative perception. This may affect funding bodies, who perceive that the public health professionals do not produce an effective intervention.

It may also be negatively perceived by the potential subject group, who may become disillusioned and believe that nutrition changes are difficult to implement and ignore any future such programmes.

This therefore emphasises the need for careful planning to maximise the chances of success (see Figure 61.2).

Food policy

The field of public health nutrition sits within the organisational framework of a national food policy. Food policy in its turn is informed by several influences (Figure 61.1), including the scientific evidence base, which comes from nutrition scientists.

Food policy is complex but its core aim is to ensure a safe, wholesome and nutritious supply of food to the population.

Included within the remit of a food policy are issues relating to agriculture, rural development, the environment and health; it is within the area of health that food safety regulations and nutrition are to be found.

Food safety is a major consideration of food policy, and with a global trade in food, legislative and regulatory requirements are frequently reviewed. Because of the high profile and immediate risk that is associated with infringements of food safety, this aspect of food policy tends to have a high priority, at the expense of nutrition policy.

However, **nutritional aspects** of food policy are relevant, as they can determine the food choices made by the population, and their nutritional consequences.

- *Guidance about food choices* is one of the key aspects of nutrition policy, usually expressed in the form of dietary guidelines. The majority of countries now use food-based dietary guidelines, represented in some form of model, either a plate, pyramid or food circle. Foods to be eaten in greatest amounts are represented by the largest segment, with foods advised in smaller amounts forming a lesser proportion of the model.

- The scientific basis of the dietary guidelines comes from the dietary requirements and reference standards that also exist in most countries.

- National nutrition policy may also incorporate **other interventions** such as:

  –fortification of specific foods, such as flour, spreading fats, baby foods;

  –recommendations on taking folate supplements when planning pregnancy;

  –advice to avoid liver, which is rich in vitamin A, when pregnant;

  –regulations regarding school meal standards.

Nutrition issues also form a part of **multiple initiatives to improve health** across the population, and currently may focus on:

- weight reduction, together with associated comorbidities such as diabetes and coronary heart disease;

- improving the diets of preschool children by attention to food in nurseries as well as programmes to help develop skills among mothers;
- improving access to health care, including better food in low-income areas;
- improving food in hospitals.

All of the above initiatives require input from nutrition scientists to translate information from the research base into practical initiatives and carry these through. Public health nutritionists are ideally placed to carry out this role. In addition dietitians possess these skills, and some therefore also work in the community in health promotion activities.

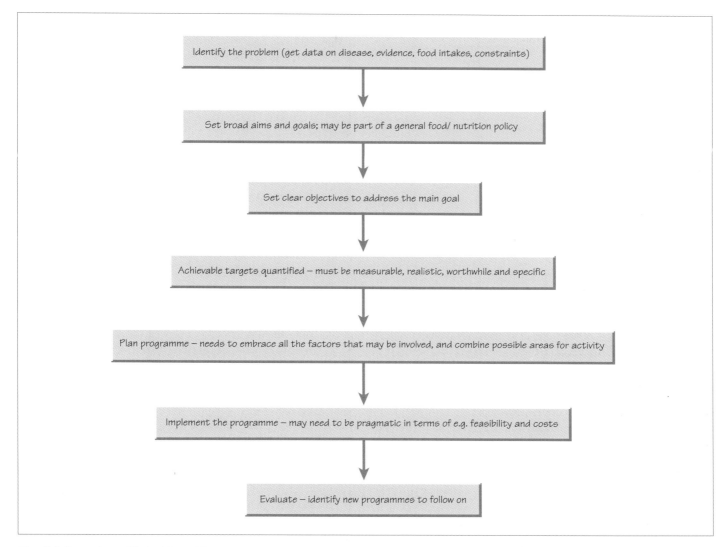

Fig. 61.2 Stages in a public health nutrition programme.

62 Promoting nutritional health: the role of the dietitian

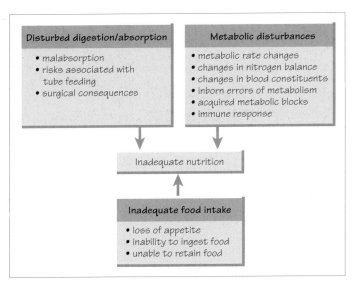

Disturbed digestion/absorption
- malabsorption
- risks associated with tube feeding
- surgical consequences

Metabolic disturbances
- metabolic rate changes
- changes in nitrogen balance
- changes in blood constituents
- inborn errors of metabolism
- acquired metabolic blocks
- immune response

Inadequate nutrition

Inadequate food intake
- loss of appetite
- inability to ingest food
- unable to retain food

Fig. 62.1 Factors contributing to inadequate nutrition that can be addressed by a dietitian.

Aims

(1) To consider the role of the dietitian in identifying and providing nutritional support for patients at risk of malnutrition.

(2) To describe the role of the dietitian in advising on dietary modifications.

(3) To identify other roles of dietitians.

Dietitians have a scientific training in diet and nutrition and are experts in translating this scientific information about food and health into practical terms that everyone can understand.

The role of dietitians varies in different countries. In the UK the majority work within the NHS, wherein most are involved in *clinical nutrition*, which is the application of nutritional science for people with a variety of medical problems. Clinical nutrition is likely to include other health professionals, such as doctors, pharmacists, biochemists and several other therapists in multidisciplinary teams.

Causes of nutritional problems

People with medical problems present a different nutritional challenge to those who are well. Avoiding malnutrition, or undernutrition, or treating it if has already happened, are the key priorities.

The three-stage model of potential threats to nutrition may be used to summarise how problems may arise (Figure 62.1).

(1) **Intake:** In healthy people this is the main area that can create problems, and is often addressed by the public health nutritionist. Medical conditions may cause additional problems, related to appetite, sickness, physical difficulties of ingestion (e.g. requiring tube feeding).

(2) **Digestion and absorption:** In healthy people, 'minor' medical problems may compromise the efficiency of these processes, for example the use of indigestion remedies, laxatives or mild food poisoning may all contribute to poor absorption. In acute or chronic

medical conditions, problems can include: malabsorption, failure of enzymic secretions, blockages or surgical consequences.

(3) **Metabolism:** Other than increased needs in growth, healthy people generally have few deficiency problems associated with metabolic changes. However, in disease, there are often major changes in metabolism, which give rise to the largest group of causes of potential deficiency that need to be addressed by clinical nutrition. For example, changes to metabolic rate, muscle wasting, blood loss, electrolyte imbalances and inflammatory states may all alter nutritional needs.

Identifying those in need of nutritional support

In order to identify the most appropriate response in any situation, it is necessary to *screen* patients and if necessary follow this up with a more in-depth nutritional *assessment*. This is discussed in Chapter 3.

Nutritional support must be timely, provided by the most appropriate route, and meet the ongoing needs of the patient. The intervention must be monitored, its effects evaluated across a number of indicators and the results documented.

Dietetic intervention in disease states

In addition to nutritional support, which may be needed in a variety of patients, the dietitian also provides advice on *modification of diets* for many chronic disease states, to improve health and quality of life. These include:

- Modification of basic healthy eating principles for the management of body weight, blood lipids and uncomplicated type 2 diabetes.
- Adjustment of the dietary content of a specific nutrient, for example fat, fibre, protein, salt, lactose or potassium, which may apply to a number of conditions.
- Exclusion of particular foods that may be the cause of specific sensitivity, such as wheat (gluten content), milk, eggs or nuts, whilst ensuring the diet remains nutritionally adequate.
- Alteration of the texture of foods to facilitate eating and swallowing.
- Providing practical advice and help for managing any dietary restrictions or modifications so they can be carried out in the home, whilst always taking into account the patient's particular situation, likes and dislikes.

Community dietetics

Dietitians also work in the community setting, where they can provide a clinical nutrition service within the primary care setting, as well as undertaking home visits to support patients.

In addition, community dietitians may take on some public health nutrition roles, providing nutrition education and health promotion to other health professionals, voluntary groups, schools and youth groups, local authorities and social services.

Sports dietitians

Sports dietitians provide specialist advice to athletes and other sports people, either on a one-to-one basis, or working with teams and

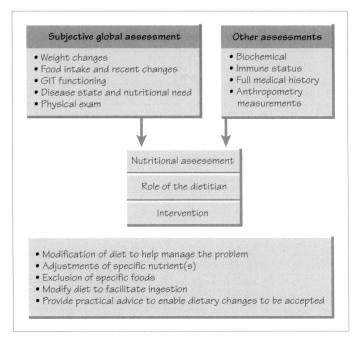

Subjective global assessment

- Weight changes
- Food intake and recent changes
- GIT functioning
- Disease state and nutritional need
- Physical exam

Other assessments

- Biochemical
- Immune status
- Full medical history
- Anthropometry measurements

Nutritional assessment

Role of the dietitian

Intervention

- Modification of diet to help manage the problem
- Adjustments of specific nutrient(s)
- Exclusion of specific foods
- Modify diet to facilitate ingestion
- Provide practical advice to enable dietary changes to be accepted

Fig. 62.2 A summary of patient assessment and routes for intervention by a dietitian.

coaches. They may also train other sports professionals who work within the leisure industry.

Dietitians in the food and pharmaceutical industry

There are a number of companies that produce special dietary products for use in clinical settings. Dietitians are involved in the development of these, using research evidence to inform new product development. They also advise hospital pharmacies and dietitians about the products that are available and their use.

Within the food industry, including the retail sector, dietitians may work on the development of new products, as well as providing consumer information about the range available. Dietitians also monitor nutritional standards for products that carry specific labelling information about suitability for people with medical conditions.

Freelance dietitians

Some dietitians provide a freelance service, using their knowledge of food and nutrition issues in the broadcast and written media including newspapers and consumer magazines, as well as providing consultancy for a range of companies and working in private practice.

Research dietitians

Underpinning the whole of dietetic practice is an evidence base that needs to be kept updated. This is the responsibility of all dietitians, who need to question and evaluate their practice. However, some dietitians work specifically in research and in this way add to the body of knowledge.

Importance of communication

The key to successfully modifying the diet of an individual is effective communication. Dietitians have to be skilled communicators, and in terms of giving dietary advice must take into consideration:

- the individual's existing food choices and the factors influencing these;
- their motivation to change;
- how to communicate this, taking into account all aspects of the communication process, including verbal and nonverbal communication, and the individual's capacity to understand the messages;
- how to change the individual's behaviour by understanding the psychological aspects of behaviour and working with these to arrive at agreed strategies and goals.

In effect, the approach and outcome with every individual may be different.

Dietitians also need to consider the ethics of their practice and recognise the limits of what they can ask people to do, and also when to stop in terms of dietary change or intervention.

Throughout all dietetic practice evaluating the outcomes of any intervention is important. This requires dietitians to be reflective and consider how their own approach has had an influence on the interaction with the patient, and to consider if in the future this can be modified for a better outcome. In addition, auditing the practice of a team of dietitians can show the overall effectiveness and indicate if changes need to be made.

The vitamins: summary of functions and food sources

Vitamin	Major functions	Food sources
Water-soluble vitamins		
Vitamin C	Reducing agent (acts as an antioxidant), reacts with free radicals. Cofactor for hydroxylase enzymes in synthesis of neurotransmitters, collagen. Promotes iron absorption	Fruits (citrus and blackcurrants especially rich), green vegetables (also peppers, tomatoes), potatoes (varies with season). Milk is a minor source
B complex group of vitamins		
Thiamin (vitamin B_1)	As thiamin diphosphate; acts as cofactor for a number of metabolic reactions, especially involved in carbohydrate metabolism. Nerve conduction	Whole cereal grains, fortified breakfast cereals and flour, beans, seeds and nuts. Pork, liver
Riboflavin (vitamin B_2)	As part of flavoprotein coenzymes, plays a key role in oxidation-reduction reactions of metabolic pathways; energy release	Milk and milk products, liver and eggs. Breakfast cereals and cereal products containing milk or eggs. Dark-green vegetables. Tea
Niacin	As part of NAD involved in energy-yielding and energy-requiring reactions. Metabolism of carbohydrates, proteins and fats	Can also be synthesised from tryptophan, so obtained from protein-containing foods. Main sources are meat (including poultry and liver), legumes, cereals, milk and dairy products, seafood, vegetables and peanuts. Some in coffee and cocoa
Pyridoxine (vitamin B_6)	Role in metabolic reactions, especially those involved with amino acid metabolism. Also involved in lipid and glycogen metabolism. Synthesis of brain neurotransmitters and porphyrin for red blood cells	Widely distributed in unprocessed foods. Whole-grain cereals, peanuts, walnuts, pulses, meat (including liver and poultry), fish, potatoes and vegetables
Folate	Transfer of single-carbon units, important in amino acid metabolism. Role in purine and pyrimidine synthesis for DNA and RNA formation	Green leafy and other vegetables, liver, fortified breakfast cereals, whole-grain cereal products, some bread, peanuts, citrus fruit and juices, potatoes. Beer and tea
Vitamin B_{12}	Cofactor for methyltransferase, closely linked to folate metabolism. Synthesis of methionine. Nerve myelination. Fatty acid metabolism	Found only in foods of animal origin: useful sources are liver, meat, eggs, milk, fish. Seaweed and algae can be a source for vegans
Pantothenic acid	Part of coenzyme A: central role in almost all metabolic reactions yielding energy	Widely distributed: meat (especially organ meats), eggs, peanuts, milk, potatoes and green leafy vegetables
Biotin	Cofactor for carboxylase enzymes, used in lipogenesis, gluconeogenesis and metabolism of branched-chain amino acids	Widely distributed: liver, eggs, peanuts, yeast, bran, vegetables, meat, fish, cereals and milk
Fat-soluble vitamins		
Vitamin A	Cell differentiation (especially epithelia and bone cells) and therefore growth, red blood cell formation, immunocompetence, part of visual pigment in retina	As retinol: in animal foods, including liver, meat, milk and dairy products, eggs, oily fish and fish oils As carotenoids: in plant foods, including green, red and orange vegetables, orange/red fruit
Vitamin D	On activation to 1,25-dihydroxycholecalciferol (calcitriol), regulates calcium absorption from the gut, calcium excretion and bone mineralisation to ensure calcium and phosphate homeostasis	Synthesised in skin on exposure to UV light Dietary sources important when UV exposure limited: oily fish and fish oils, liver, eggs and dairy products, meat. Fortified products: margarine, breakfast cereals, milk-based drinks, baby foods
Vitamin E	Antioxidant role in lipid environments; contributes to integrity, stability and function of cellular membranes	Vegetable oils, whole cereals and their products, green leafy vegetables, nuts and seeds Poultry, fish and eggs
Vitamin K	Gamma-carboxylation of glutamic acid residues, used in blood clotting and bone mineralisation	Vegetable oils, and their products; green leafy vegetables and peas. Liver. Tea

The minerals: summary of functions and food sources

Mineral	Functions	Food sources
Calcium	Major component of bone; provides strength and density. Ionic calcium in body fluids needed for blood clotting and nerve/muscle function. Activates enzymes within cells and needed for release of some hormones	Milk and dairy products. Fortified soya milk, green leafy vegetables; fish with small bones; nuts and seeds. Dried fruit, watercress and black treacle. Fortified flour and its products. Hard water
Phosphorus	Principally found in bone, but also distributed throughout all tissues of the body. Essential in metabolism as part of ATP, a component of DNA and RNA and as buffer in body fluids	Present in most foodstuffs, although whole-grain cereals and legumes may contain insoluble forms, difficult to absorb. Meat, poultry, fish, eggs and dairy products are useful sources. Also used as an additive in bakery goods, processed meats and soft drinks
Sodium	Major extracellular cation, also found in bone. Key role in water balance, nerve conduction and active transport across cell membranes. Regulated by several hormones, including angiotensin and aldosterone, and by renal excretion	Natural food sources, especially plant foods, contain low levels of sodium. Food preparation and processing add sodium to the diet, during cooking, as a preservative, flavouring agents and texture enhancer. Inclusion of processed foods in the diet raises sodium intakes by varying amounts
Potassium	Major intracellular ion, predominantly bound to protein and phosphate. Essential for fluid, electrolyte and acid–base balance, nerve impulse propagation and muscle contraction. Regulated by hormonal action and renal excretion	Widely distributed in food, especially of plant origin; rich sources include bananas, kiwi fruit, avocado, potato and spinach. Cereals and dairy products may be useful if eaten regularly. Meat and fish are important dietary sources. Processed foods are often low in potassium
Magnesium	Found in the skeleton and soft tissues, and almost entirely intracellular. Involved in the development and maintenance of bone, and in the activity of many enzyme reactions in metabolism, where it stabilises the binding to substrates	High levels of magnesium found in: whole grains, legumes, nuts, seafood and green leafy vegetables. Moderate levels occur in fruit and dairy products. Refined and processed foods are low in magnesium
Iron	Transport of oxygen within the haemoglobin molecule. Also found in myoglobin to provide oxygen in muscle. Functions as part of several enzyme systems, critical for energy production, as well as within the immune system. A key property is the ability to switch between the oxidised and reduced states	Found in meat, fish and eggs; liver is a very rich source. Haemoglobin and myoglobin in these provide haem iron, which is well absorbed. Non-haem iron occurs principally in foods of plant origin: cereals, legumes and vegetables. Absorption is poorer from these sources, and strongly affected by other dietary components
Zinc	Widely distributed in the body; zinc has a catalytic, structural and regulatory role. It is involved in enzymes that have a role in metabolism of macronutrients, production of energy, gene transcription, transport of gases and antioxidant systems. Immune system function	Found in protein-containing foods, such as meat, seafoods and dairy products. Cereals and legumes are potentially good sources, although bioavailability may be low due to the presence of phytate. Fruit and leafy vegetables are low in zinc
Copper	Plays a role in the utilisation of iron; required for the synthesis of neurotransmitters, production of ATP, formation of collagen, acute response to infection and antioxidant roles	Main contributors in the diet are meat, meat products and cereal products. Rich sources include liver, shellfish, nuts and seeds, legumes and whole cereal grains. Bananas, potatoes, tomatoes and mushrooms are intermediate sources
Selenium	A component of glutathione peroxidase, an important antioxidant in the body; role in the function of immune system. Interaction with vitamin E	Selenium content of foods varies with the soil levels, and is related to the protein content. Brazil nuts are a rich source; meat, eggs, cereals, dairy products and fish contribute selenium in the overall diet
Iodine	As iodide, required for synthesis of thyroid hormones, which regulate development and metabolism	Seafoods, including seaweed, are a rich source; milk is a source from iodide compounds in the dairy industry. Bakery goods contain iodide from flour improvers
Fluoride	Incorporated into apatite, forms fluoroapatite, which increases the hardness of teeth, and resistance to caries	Present in water at varying concentrations. May be added in fluoridation. Also found in tea and seafoods
Chromium	As a component of glucose-tolerance factor, potentiates action of insulin. May also be involved in lipid metabolism	Content is very variable: rich sources are spices, yeast, beef, whole grains, legumes, dried fruit and nuts. Refined foods have a low content

Department of Health Report on Health and Social Subjects: Dietary reference values for food energy and nutrients for the United Kingdom

Report of the Panel on Dietary Reference Values of the Committee on Medical Aspects of Food Policy

All material reproduced from this report is Crown copyright and is reproduced with the permission of the Controller of HMSO.

Table 1 Estimated average requirements (EARs) for energy.

Age	EARs MJ/d (kcal/d)	
	Males	**Females**
0–3 months	2.28 (545)	2.16 (515)
4–6 months	2.89 (690)	2.69 (645)
7–9 months	3.44 (625)	3.20 (765)
10–12 months	3.85 (920)	3.61 (865)
1–3 years	5.15 (1230)	4.86 (1165)
4–6 years	7.16 (1715)	6.46 (1545)
7–10 years	8.24 (1970)	7.28 (1740)
11–14 years	9.27 (2220)	7.72 (1845)
15–18 years	11.51 (2755)	8.83 (2110)
19–50 years	10.60 (2550)	8.10 (1940)
51–59 years	10.60 (2550)	8.00 (1900)
60–64 years	9.93 (2380)	7.99 (1900)
65–74 years	9.71 (2330)	7.96 (1900)
75 + years	8.77 (2100)	7.61 (1810)
Pregnancy		+0.80[a] (200)
Lactation:		
1 month		+1.90 (450)
2 months		+2.20 (530)
3 months		+2.40 (570)
4–6 months (Group 1)		+2.00 (480)
4–6 months (Group 2)		+2.40 (570)
>6 months (Group 1)		+1.00 (240)
>6 months (Group 2)		+2.30 (550)

[a] Last trimester only

Summary tables

The following tables set out in summary form the findings of the Panel:

Estimated average requirements for energy	Table 1
Dietary reference values for fat and carbohydrate	Table 2
Reference nutrient intakes for protein	Table 3
Reference nutrient intakes for vitamins	Table 4
Reference nutrient intakes for minerals	Table 5
Safe intakes	Table 6

Table 2 Dietary reference values for fat and carbohydrate for adults as a percentage of daily total energy intake (percentage of food energy).

	Individual minimum	Population average	Individual maximum
Saturated fatty acids		10 (11)	
Cis-polyunsaturated fatty acids		6 (6.5)	10
n3	0.2		
n6	1.0		
Cis-monounsaturated fatty acids		12 (13)	
Trans fatty acids		2 (2)	
Total fatty acids		30 (32.5)	
Total fat		**33 (35)**	
Non-milk extrinsic sugars	0	10 (11)	
Intrinsic and milk sugars and starch		37 (39)	
Total carbohydrate		**47 (50)**	
Non-starch polysaccharide (g/d)	**12**	**18**	**24**

The average percentage contribution to total energy does not total 100% because figures for protein and alcohol are excluded. Protein intakes average 15 per cent of total energy, which is above the RNI. It is recognised that many individuals will derive some energy from alcohol, and this has been assumed to average 5 per cent approximating current intakes. However, the Panel allowed that some groups might not drink alcohol and that for some purposes nutrient intakes as a proportion of food energy (without alcohol) might be useful. Therefore average figures are given as percentages both of total energy and, in parenthesis, of food energy.

Table 3 Reference nutrient intakes for protein.

Age	Reference nutrient intakes[a] g/d
0–3 months	12.5[b]
4–6 months	12.7
7–9 months	13.7
10–12 months	14.9
1–3 years	14.5
4–6 years	19.7
7–10 years	28.3
Males:	
11–14 years	42.1
15–18 years	55.2
19–50 years	55.3
50+ years	53.5
Females:	
11–14 years	41.2
15–18 years	45.0
19–50 years	45.0
50+ years	46.5
Pregnancy[c]	+6
Lactation:[c]	
0–4 months	+11
4+ months	+8

[a] These figures, based on egg and milk protein, assume complete digestibility.

[b] No values for infants 0–3 months are given by WHO. The RNI is calculated from the recommendations of COMA.

[c] To be added to adult requirement through all stages of pregnancy and lactation.

Table 4 Reference nutrient intakes for vitamins.

Age	Thiamin mg/d	Riboflavin mg/d	Niacin (nicotinic acid equivalent) mg/d[†]	Vitamin B$_6$ mg/d	Vitamin B$_{12}$ µg/d	Folate µg/d	Vitamin C mg/d	Vitamin A µg/d	Vitamin D µg/d
0–3 months	0.2	0.4	3	0.2	0.3	50	25	350	8.5
4–6 months	0.2	0.4	3	0.2	0.3	5-	25	350	8.5
7–9 months	0.2	0.4	4	0.3	0.4	50	25	350	7
10–12 months	0.3	0.4	5	0.4	0.4	50	25	350	7
1–3 years	0.5	0.6	8	0.7	0.5	70	30	400	7
4–6 years	0.7	0.8	11	0.9	0.8	100	30	400	—
7–10 years	0.7	1.0	12	1.0	1.0	150	30	500	—
Males									
11–14 years	0.9	1.2	15	1.2	1.2	200	35	600	—
15–18 years	1.1	1.3	18	1.5	1.5	200	40	700	—
19–50 years	1.0	1.3	17	1.4	1.5	200	40	700	—
50+ years	0.9	1.3	16	1.4	1.5	200	40	700	**
Females									
11–14 years	0.7	1.1	12	1.0	1.2	200	35	600	—
15–18 years	0.8	1.1	14	1.2	1.5	200	40	600	—
19–50 years	0.8	1.1	13	1.2	1.5	200	40	600	—
50+ years	0.8	1.1	12	1.2	1.5	200	40	600	**
Pregnancy	+0.1***	+0.3	*	*	*	+100	+10***	+100	10
Lactation:									
0-4 months	+0.2	+0.5	+2	*	+0.5	+60	+30	+350	10
4+ months	+0.2	+0.5	+2	*	+0.5	+60	+30	+350	10

* No increment.

** After age 65 the RNI is 10 µg/d for men and women.

*** For last trimester only.

[†] Based on protein providing 14.7 per cent of EAR for energy.

Table 5 Reference nutrient intakes for minerals.

Age	Calcium mg/d	Phosphorus[a] mg/d	Magnesium mg/d	Sodium mg/d[b]	Potassium mg/d[c]	Chloride[d] mg/d	Iron mg/d	Zinc mg/d	Copper mg/d	Selenium μg/d	Iodine μg/d
0–3 months	525	400	55	210	800	320	1.7	4.0	0.2	10	50
4–6 months	525	400	60	280	850	400	4.3	4.0	0.3	13	60
7–9 months	525	400	75	320	700	500	7.8	5.0	0.3	10	60
10–12 months	525	400	80	350	700	500	7.8	5.0	0.3	10	60
1–3 years	350	270	85	500	800	800	6.9	5.0	0.4	15	70
4–6 years	450	350	120	700	1100	1100	6.1	6.5	0.6	20	100
7–10 years	550	450	200	1200	2000	1800	8.7	7.0	0.7	30	110
Males											
11–14 years	1000	775	280	1600	3100	2500	11.3	9.0	0.8	45	130
15–18 years	1000	775	300	1600	3500	2500	11.3	9.5	1.0	70	140
19–50 years	700	550	300	1600	3500	2500	8.7	9.5	1.2	75	140
50+ years	700	550	300	1600	3500	2500	8.7	9.5	1.2	75	140
Females											
11–14 years	800	625	280	1600	3100	2500	14.8[e]	9.0	0.8	45	130
15–18 years	800	625	300	1600	3500	2500	14.8[e]	7.0	1.0	60	140
19–50 years	700	550	270	1600	3500	2500	14.8[e]	7.0	1.2	60	140
50+ years	700	550	270	1600	3500	2500	8.7	7.0	1.2	60	140
Pregnancy	*	*	*	*	*	*	*	*	*	*	*
Lactation:											
0-4 months	+550	+440	+50	*	*	*	*	+6.0	+0.3	+15	*
4+ months	+550	+440	+50	*	*	*	*	+2.5	+0.3	+15	*

* No increment.

[a] Phosphorus RNI is set equal to calcium in molar terms.

[b] 1 mmol sodium = 23 mg.

[c] 1 mmol potassium = 39 mg.

[d] Corresponds to sodium 1 mmol.

[e] Insufficient for women with high menstrual losses where the most practical way of meeting iron requirements is to take iron supplements.

Table 6 Safe intakes.

Nutrient	Safe intake
Vitamins:	
Pantothenic acid	
Adults	3–7 mg/d
Infants	1.7 mg/d
Biotin	10–200 µg/d
Vitamin E	
Men	above 4 mg/d
Women	above 3 mg/d
Children	0.4 mg/g polyunsaturated fatty acids
Vitamin K	
Adults	1 µg/kg/d
Infants	10 µg/d
Minerals:	
Manganese	
Adults	above 1.4 mg (26 µmol)/d
Infants, children and adolescents	above 16 µg (0.3 µmol)/d
Molybdenum	
Adults	50–400 µg/d
Infants, children and adolescents	0.5–1.5 µg/kg/d
Chromium	
Adults	above 25 µg (0.5 µmol)/d
Children and adolescents	0.1–1.0 µg 2–20 nmol)/kg/d
Fluoride	
Children over 6 years and adults	0.5 mg/kg/d (3 µmol/kg/day)
Children over 6 months	0.12 mg/kg/d (6 µmol/kg/day)
Infants under 6 months	0.22 mg/kg/d (12 µmol/kg/day)

Table 7 Energy expenditure of various activities of moderate duration grouped according to Physical Activity (PAR).

PAR 1.2 (1.0 to 1.4)

Lying at rest:	Reading
Sitting at rest:	Watching TV; reading; writing; calculating; playing cards; listening to radio; eating
Standing at rest	

PAR 1.6 (1.5 to 1.8)

Sitting:	Sewing; knitting; playing piano; driving
Standing:	Preparing vegetables; washing dishes; ironing; general office and laboratory work

PAR 2.1 (1.9 to 2.4)

Standing:	Mixed household chores (dusting and cleaning); washing small clothes; cooking activities; hairdressing; playing snooker; bowling

PAR 2.8 (2.5 to 3.3)

Standing:	Dressing and undressing; showering; 'hoovering'; making beds
Walking:	3–4 km/h; playing cricket
Industrial:	Tailoring; shoemaking; electrical; machine tool; painting and decorating

PAR 3.7 (3.4 to 4.4)

Standing:	Mopping floor; gardening; cleaning windows; playing table tennis; sailing
Walking:	4–6 km/h; golf
Industrial:	Motor vehicle repairs; carpentry, chemical; joinery; bricklaying

PAR 4.8 (4.5 to 4.9)

Standing:	Polishing furniture; chopping wood; heavy gardening; volley ball
Walking:	6–7 km/h
Exercise:	Dancing; moderate swimming; gentle cycling; slow jogging
Occupational:	Labouring; hoeing; road construction; digging and shovelling; felling trees

PAR 6.9 (6.0 to 7.9)

Wallking:	Uphill with load or cross-country; climbing stairs
Exercise:	Average jogging; cycling
Sports:	Football; more energetic swimming; tennis; skiing

Glossary

AOAC (Association of Official Analytical Chemists) method for analysis of dietary fibre: A method that uses an enzymatic/gravimetric process that includes lignin and resistant starch in the analysis.

Appetite: A desire to eat a specific food, or a type of food (cf. hunger).

Basal metabolic rate (BMR): The minimum amount of energy expended by the body to maintain life in the awake state. It is measured under strict conditions.

Bias: The deviation of results from the true situation, and may be applied to processes that lead to such deviation. These may include aspects of study design, performance or interpretation that lead to inferences that deviate from the true situation.

Biological Value (BV): A measure of protein quality that takes into account the digestibility of protein by comparing nitrogen retention against nitrogen absorption.

Body Mass Index: An index calculated from the subject's body weight (in kilograms), divided by the square of the height (in metres). This is widely used to indicate categories for underweight, normal weight, overweight and obesity.

Brown adipose tissue (BAT): A type of adipose tissue, found principally in young mammals, highly metabolically active and thermogenic when stimulated. It contains more mitochondria, blood capillaries and nerve fibres than the more prevalent white adipose tissue.

Cardiovascular disease (CVD): A general term for the presence of atherosclerosis, a narrowing and hardening of the arteries, which affects the flow of blood within them. There is an increased risk of inadequate delivery of oxygen to meet the demand for exercise (resulting in pain on exertion), or a blockage to the blood flow, which may result in a failure of function in the affected area, for example in the heart or brain.

CETP: (cholesterol ester transfer protein) A protein that enables HDLs to transfer cholesterol esters into VLDLs and chylomicrons for transport to the liver, in exchange for TAGs. Such transfer in large amounts results in 'dense HDL', which are more atherogenic.

CCK (cholecystokinin): A hormone released in the gut that stimulates the secretion of bile. It can also act as a satiety signal, and may be found in the brain.

CHO: Abbreviation commonly used for carbohydrates.

COMA: Committee on Medical Aspects of Food and Nutrition Policy. In the UK, formerly, it produced reports on nutrition issues for the Department of Health. It has now been replaced by the Scientific Advisory Committee on Nutrition (SACN).

Confounding: The possibility that a variable affects the outcome of interest, by being associated with the factor under investigation.

Coronary heart disease (CHD): One of the manifestations of the process of atherosclerosis, which results in narrowing of the coronary arteries. Symptoms may include angina (chest pain on exertion). Blockage of a narrowed vessel may result in a heart attack (myocardial infarction). The outcome will depend on the extent of the affected heart tissue.

CRP: C-reactive protein, a marker of inflammation released by the liver. One of the acute-phase proteins.

Demispan: A surrogate measure for height. Can be taken in a seated subject, and measures the distance from the tip of the middle finger on the right-hand side to the centre of the sternal notch. Prediction equations to obtain height from this measurement are available for men and women of different ages.

DHA (docosahexaenoic acid): A fatty acid with 22 carbon atoms and six double bonds, and a member of the *n*-3 family. Found predominantly in oily fish.

Digestible energy: The energy theoretically obtainable from a food, after allowing for losses during digestion and absorption.

Direct calorimetry: The use of an insulated chamber to measure the heat (and therefore energy) output from a subject over a period of time. The method was used in classical studies to establish the basic theory of energy exchanges. Used infrequently at present, due to costs, technical demands and limitations of activity that can be performed by the subject.

Diverticular disease: A condition characterised by the presence of pouches of mucosal lining protruding through the various layers of the bowel wall, which may eventually extrude from the outside surface. These are predominantly in the sigmoid colon. Generally asymptomatic in the majority of patients. Pain in the lower left quadrant of the abdomen may be confused with irritable bowel syndrome. Epidemiological evidence suggests an association with low levels of dietary fibre intake.

Doubly-labelled water technique (DLW): A method for the measurement of energy expenditure that involves the consumption of a small amount of water with labelled hydrogen and oxygen. The excretion of the radioactive label over a period of time (7 or 14 days) is used to calculate metabolic activity and thus energy expenditure.

DRV (Dietary Reference Values): A general term covering all UK dietary standards. It includes RNI (Reference Nutrient Intake), EAR (Estimated Average Requirement) and LRNI (Lower Reference Nutrient Intake). In other countries similar values may have alternative names, for example Recommended Daily Amounts (RDA).

Energy density: A measure of the amount of energy supplied in a food, expressed per unit weight. Lower energy density foods are generally dilute, containing a large amount of water, or non-nutritional factors such as non-digestible carbohydrate. Foods with high energy density contain a large amount of energy in a relatively small volume, and are likely to be rich in fat, or low in water content.

EPA (eicosapentaenoic acid): A fatty acid with 20 carbons and five double bonds, a member of the *n*-3 family. Found predominantly in oily fish. Some conversion to DHA can occur in the body.

Food fortification: The addition of a nutrient or nutrients to a widely consumed food in order to improve the nutritional intake in a population. Fortification may be legally required or occur on a voluntary basis at the discretion of a manufacturer.

Food security: Access by all to a safe and affordable food supply that is of a nutritional quality to meet the needs for physical and mental development and healthy and productive lives.

Functional foods: Products that carry a claim of health-promoting properties, usually on the basis of an added ingredient, which may or may not be naturally present in the food. Claims that can be made are controlled by law.

GDA (Guideline Daily Amount): An average recommended level of intake for a particular nutrient, calculated from the Dietary Reference Values, for a 'typical' man and woman aged 19–50 years. For men the GDA for energy is 2500 kcal, for women, it is 2000 kcal. The fat, saturated fat, carbohydrate and sugars levels are calculated from the DRV values. Salt levels are based on the current recommendation by SACN (6 g/day). They are principally used in food labelling.

Glycaemic Index (GI): A ratio describing the ability of a carbohydrate to raise levels of blood glucose, in comparison with the increase obtained following a standard glucose dose. Foods with a high GI raise glucose levels rapidly, whereas those with a low GI have a small effect on blood glucose levels.

Gross energy: The energy contained in a food, as measured by combustion in a bomb calorimeter.

High-density lipoprotein (HDL): One of the aggregate particles used to transport lipids in the circulation. Sometimes termed a 'good' lipoprotein because of an association of elevated HDL levels with lower risk of CHD.

HMGCoA-reductase (3-hydroxy-3-methylglutaryl CoA reductase): An enzyme used in the synthesis of cholesterol.

Hunger: A state of motivation to eat, associated with an internal state of energy depletion.

Iodine deficiency disorder (IDD): One of the three commonest nutritional deficiencies worldwide. It is associated with inadequate supply of iodine in the food chain in a geographical area. May affect infants and women particularly.

Iron deficiency anaemia (IDA): One of the three commonest nutritional deficiencies worldwide. Attributable to low iron intakes and high requirements. Affects particularly children and women of childbearing age, especially in pregnancy. Results in debility and tiredness, poor growth and physical and cognitive development. Severe anaemia may result in death of pregnant women.

Incidence: The proportion of new cases of a condition that occur in a population during a particular period of time. Thus incidence is calculated as new cases/population at risk.

Indirect calorimetry: An experimental approach that utilises measurement of the flux of respiratory gases to obtain values for energy expenditure. Short-term measurements may use portable or stationary gas-collecting or monitoring devices, such as Douglas bags, ventilated hoods and respirometers. The most useful method is the doubly-labelled water (DLW) technique, which uses stable isotopes of oxygen and hydrogen, administered as water. The differential rates of elimination of the two isotopes provide information about the flux of carbon dioxide and oxygen and thereby heat production. Diet records may also be kept to monitor the proportions of macronutrients being consumed in the diet.

LCAT (lecithin-cholesterol acyl transferase): An enzyme involved in the synthesis of cholesterol esters from cholesterol, which allows concentration gradients for uptake of cholesterol to be maintained.

Lipoprotein lipase (LPL): The enzyme found on the endothelial surfaces of muscle and adipose tissue that breaks down TAGs in circulating VLDLs and chylomicrons and allows uptake of fatty acids into storage sites or for use in active tissue.

Low birth weight (LBW): Generally used to describe a newborn who weighs less than 2.5 kg.

Low-density lipoprotein (LDL): One of the aggregate particles used to transport lipids in the circulation. A major carrier of cholesterol, and sometimes considered a 'bad' lipoprotein because of an association of raised LDL levels with greater risk of CHD.

MAC (mid-arm circumference): A measurement of the circumference of the upper arm, taken at the midpoint between shoulder and elbow. When used in conjunction with fat measurement by skinfold thickness, can be used to calculate mid-arm muscle circumference, which is used as an indicator of degree of undernutrition.

Mediterranean diet: A term used to describe a traditional food intake pattern, characterised by large amounts of fruit and vegetables, bread or other starchy staple, olive oil and dairy produce, with small amounts of meat and fish. This has been associated with lower incidence of NR-NCDs.

Metabolisable energy: The energy provided by a food during its biochemical transformation. This value is normally calculated by the use of 'proximate principles', and is the value for energy content that appears in tables of food composition.

Monounsaturated fatty acid (MUFA): A fatty acid that contains one double bond in the chain. Oleic acid (C18) is considered to be the most important member of this group, and a key component of the Mediterranean diet.

Morbidity: The occurrence of disease (usually expressed over a period of time to give a morbidity rate).

Mortality: The occurrence of death (usually expressed over a period of time, to give a mortality rate).

Net protein utilisation (NPU): One of the ways in which protein quality has been assessed. NPU is a measure of the retention of nitrogen in relation to the intake.

Neural tube defects (NTD): A group of birth defects in which the brain, spinal cord, skull and vertebral column fail to develop properly, leading to conditions such as spina bifida and anencephaly.

Non-esterified fatty acids (NEFAs): (or free fatty acids) The fatty acids that are generally released from breakdown of TAG.

Non-starch polysaccharides (NSP): A term used to describe a major fraction of the dietary fibre in the diet; includes all cellulosic and non-cellulosic polysaccharides, but excludes resistant starch. NSP values are obtained by the Englyst method of analysis.

Nutrition-related non-communicable diseases (NR-NCDs): Diseases associated with overnutrition and poorly balanced diets, with multifactorial aetiologies, such as coronary heart disease, type 2 diabetes and cancers. Previously termed 'diseases of affluence'.

Nutrition transition: A period of time when changes are occurring to nutritional supplies, such that food shortages and undernutrition are diminishing, but new diseases associated with unbalanced diets are beginning to emerge.

Peripheral vascular disease (PVD): An aspect of CVD, affecting the peripheral blood vessels.

Physical Activity Level (PAL): The average level of energy expenditure, in relation to BMR, expressed over a period of time, usually a day, or averaged over a week. PAL values of 1.4 are considered to indicate a sedentary lifestyle, values of 1.8 are recommended for protection against obesity. Individuals with physically active occupations and lifestyles tend to have PAL values above 1.75.

Physical Activity Ratio (PAR): An indicator of the metabolic cost of an activity, represented as a multiple of BMR.

PKU (phenylketonuria): One of a number of 'inborn errors of metabolism' where the absence of an enzyme or a defect in a particular metabolic pathway results in the inability to metabolise specific compounds. In the case of PKU, phenylalanine hydroxylase is absent, with the result that high levels of phenylalanine accumulate in the body, resulting in cerebral damage. Exclusion of phenylalanine from the diet is necessary.

Polyunsaturated fatty acids (PUFAs): Fatty acids that contain two or more double bonds in the molecule. The location of the double bonds characterises the 'family' to which the fatty acid belongs; those of particular relevance in nutrition are the *n*-3 and *n*-6 families, identified by the position of the first double bond, when counted from the CH_3 end of the molecule. The hydrogen atoms are arranged in *cis*- formation around double bonds in naturally occurring PUFAs.

Prevalence: The number of cases of a disease at a particular point in time. This includes all cases, and is calculated as the total cases/total population.

RBC: Abbreviation for red blood cells, i.e. erythrocytes.

Reactive oxygen species (ROS): (or oxygen-derived radicals) Part of the group of free radicals formed in the body as a result of metabolic reactions, defence mechanisms and exposure to environmental factors. A number of antioxidant systems are in place within the body to inactivate these molecules and protect against damage. They include nutrient-dependent pathways.

Resting metabolic rate (RMR): Often used interchangeably with BMR; measured under conditions that are less strict, allows inclusion of recent food intake.

Risk factor: A characteristic that is related to the subsequent occurrence of disease, e.g. cardiovascular disease. Evidence is needed to establish causality. Risk factors may interact or be independent.

Risk marker: A characteristic that is associated with the occurrence of, e.g., cardiovascular disease; it is likely to be an indicator of a lifestyle or behavioural trait, but is not causally related.

Satiation: A state of fullness that leads to the termination of eating and reduction of meal size.

Satiety: A state of post-meal repletion that delays the onset of the subsequent meal.

Saturated fatty acids (SFAs): Fatty acids that contain the maximum number of hydrogen atoms on each carbon. Fats containing a high proportion of SFAs tend to be solid at room temperature.

Short-chain fatty acids (SCFAs): These include acetic, butyric and propionic acids, which are produced in the large intestine by the fermentation of undigested carbohydrate residues, mainly resistant starch and soluble NSP. These fatty acids may be beneficial to health.

Small for gestational age (SGA): A newborn whose birth weight is lower than expected for its calculated age at delivery. These babies are considered to have experienced intrauterine growth retardation (IUGR).

Small intestine (SI): The region of the gastrointestinal tract that includes the duodenum, jejunum and ileum and lies between the stomach and the large intestine. A major site for digestion and absorption of nutrients.

TAGs (triacylglycerols; or triglycerides): A type of fat found in the diet and the body, comprising a glycerol backbone with three fatty acid molecules attached.

Taste: Physiologically, refers to the four basic tastes: sweet, sour, salt and bitter, but can also encompass food aroma and texture, as well as its hedonic or pleasure components.

Total energy expenditure (TEE): A measured, or calculated value for the amount of energy used by an individual over a 24-hour period. This may be obtained by an activity diary, or may be measured using the doubly-labelled water technique (DLW). The ratio of TEE to BMR over 24 hours gives the Physical Activity Level (PAL), which is a useful indicator of overall activity.

Trans fatty acids (TFAs): Fatty acids, generally containing several double bonds, in which the hydrogen atoms are arranged in *trans* formation around the double bonds. Some TFAs are produced by rumen bacteria and occur naturally in products from ruminant animals. Hydrogenation of fats in food processing results in formation of TFAs. They are considered potentially harmful to health.

VAD (vitamin A deficiency): One of the three commonest nutrient deficiencies worldwide. Affects resistance to infection and thus results in increased morbidity and mortality from common diseases; also results in night blindness, anaemia and eventual blindness.

Very low-density lipoprotein (VLDL): One of the aggregate particles used to transport lipids in the circulation. VLDLs carry mainly TAGs, and their persistence in the circulation is considered to be potentially atherogenic.

WBC: Abbreviation for white blood cells, or leucocytes.

Waist-to-hip ratio (WHR): A ratio of the circumference at the waist, divided by the circumference at the largest part of the hips. The ratio is generally higher in men than women; a higher ratio may be associated with 'central obesity' and is considered to be a risk factor for disease, such as diabetes.

Index